Cocaine Addiction

Other books by Arnold M. Washton

Cocaine: A Clinician's Handbook (with M. S. Gold)

Willpower's Not Enough (with D. Boundy)

Cocaine and Crack: What You Need To Know (with D. Boundy)

COCAINE ADDICTION

Treatment, Recovery, and Relapse Prevention

Arnold M. Washton, Ph.D.

W. W. NORTON & COMPANY • NEW YORK • LONDON

Certain portions of the case descriptions and accompanying quotations presented in this book have been altered, where necessary, to protect identities.

Copyright © 1989 by Arnold Washton

All rights reserved.

Printed in the United States of America.

First published as a Norton paperback 1991

Library of Congress Cataloging-in-Publication Data

Washton, Arnold M.
    Cocaine addiction : treatment, recovery, and relapse prevention /
Arnold M. Washton.–1st ed.
    p. cm.
"A Norton professional book."
Bibliography: p.
    1. Cocaine habit–Treatment.   2. Cocaine habit–Relapse-
Prevention.   I. Title.
    [DNLM: 1. Cocaine.   2. Substance Dependence–therapy.   WM 280
W319c]
RC568.C6W37   1989
616.86'3–dc19
DNLM/DLC   88-39391
for Library of Congress   CIP

ISBN 0-393-30715-8

W.W. Norton & Company, Inc., 500 Fifth Avenue, New York, N.Y. 10110
W.W. Norton & Company Ltd., 10 Coptic Street, London WC1A 1PU

0

To my wife, Nannette, and to my daughters, Tala and
Danae, for their encouragement, love, and
understanding.

Acknowledgments

FIRST AND FOREMOST, I am grateful to Nannette Stone—my wife, colleague, and personal editor—who inspired me to undertake the task of writing this book. Even before writing her own book on the subject (*Cocaine: Seduction and Solution*, Clarkson N. Potter, 1984) she had been encouraging me to write down my experiences and ideas about treating cocaine addiction in the form of a book. I finally took her advice.

My daughters, Tala and Danae, sacrificed more than a few evenings and weekends during the summer of 1988 while I remained glued to the word processor. I am grateful for their patience, understanding, and willingness to tolerate my intermittent workaholism. I promise not to spend next summer writing another book.

My special thanks go also to Donna Boundy for helping to transform this project from an idea into a reality.

Last but not least, I am grateful to the countless addicted individuals whose sufferings and triumphs have provided much of the raw material for this book. They have helped me to help others. It is my hope that the information contained in this book will contribute to increased understanding and improved treatment options for people addicted to cocaine or other mood-altering drugs.

Contents

Cocaine Addiction

Introduction

IN 1982, WHILE TREATING hard-core heroin addicts at a public clinic in Harlem, I began receiving telephone calls from desperate people who had never tried heroin, used needles, or been arrested for a crime. These callers did not resemble the Harlem addicts at all. They were typically white, employed, middle-class people in their 20s or 30s who had good jobs, good incomes, intact families, and no prior history of drug addiction or psychiatric illness. Some were high-level executives, professionals, or entrepreneurs. Most were "baby-boomers" who had used drugs occasionally or "recreationally" since late adolescence. They never thought they could become addicted, but now they had a serious problem: they were snorting cocaine, could not stop, and could not find professional help. It was well-known that cocaine was not addictive (some medical experts went so far as to liken the addiction potential of cocaine to that of peanuts or potato chips — hard to stop after taking just one), and while these callers didn't experience any withdrawal from cocaine, using it was no longer a choice for them, it was an obsession. They knew scores of other people who were using the drug and scores who seemed well on their way to becoming addicted to it.

These people felt foolish and crazy for getting addicted to a drug that was supposedly nonaddictive. They were baffled and didn't know where to turn for help. How could they find treatment when no one (including medical experts) really believed that cocaine was addictive and no treatment was

1

available? Some had gone to private therapists, but then, as now, few therapists had formal training or adequate experience in treating substance abusers. The therapists, in most cases, didn't deal directly with the drug problem; rather they sought to engage these patients in exploratory psychotherapy, hoping that resolution of underlying psychological problems would eventually resolve the drug problem. But it wasn't working. Some prescribed addictive drugs such as tranquilizers or sleeping pills, which only compounded the patient's cocaine problem. Some refused to provide any treatment whatsoever, feeling perhaps uncomfortable, frightened, or just ill-prepared to deal with substance-abusing patients.

Not only treatment professionals, but most people in the general population were unaware of how widespread cocaine use had become. Even fewer were aware of the growing numbers of cocaine users who were turning into cocaine addicts. Not a single alcohol or drug abuse treatment program in New York City at the time had a cocaine-specific treatment track, nor were these programs attempting to reach out to this growing subgroup of drug abusers.

That was the scene in late 1982, when I established the first telephone "helpline" in the U.S. for cocaine users and their families. Within two months, this local helpline was receiving over 100 calls per day as word about it spread rapidly throughout the New York metropolitan area as a result of public service announcements on local radio and television stations. In addition to exposing the enormous unmet need for accurate information about cocaine and for treatment of cocaine addiction, the helpline provided a unique opportunity to collect valuable research data during telephone interviews with randomly selected callers. These studies provided dramatic new evidence that cocaine was truly addictive and that use of the drug was rampant among the middle class. Most callers said that they felt unable to control their use, had failed repeatedly to stop using it on their own, and were often riddled with cravings and urges for the drug. Most earned over $25,000 per year and were spending over $600 per week for cocaine. They complained of numerous cocaine-related problems, including depression, paranoia, loss of sex drive, panic anxiety, headaches, sinus infections, physical and mental exhaustion, weight loss, memory problems, financial problems, family problems, and job problems. Many had turned increasingly to other drugs — alcohol, tranquilizers, sleeping pills, even heroin — to alleviate the intolerable "crash" and other aftereffects of heavy cocaine use. Some had experienced seizures or become suicidal.

These early helpline experiences caught the attention of both local and national media. Before long I was appearing on talk shows and news programs and being interviewed by newspaper and magazine reporters who were eager to disseminate the dramatic revelations about cocaine snorters who had become addicted to the drug and about the apparent epidemic of cocaine use among the middle-class. As word about the helpline spread across the country, many people far outside New York began calling for help, indicating that cocaine problems existed in many different parts of the country, not just in New York City. This fact became even more evident during my subsequent involvement with the "800-COCAINE" hotline, which at times received over 2,000 calls a day from areas all across the nation.

Since that time, within the span of only a few short years, cocaine use has become recognized as a nationwide epidemic and the drug is now almost universally considered highly dangerous and addictive. Use has spread increasingly to women, minority groups, lower-income groups, and adolescents. Cocaine has infiltrated virtually every large city as well as many suburbs and small towns across the country. Once called the "champagne of drugs" and the "rich man's high," cocaine has now become an "equal opportunity drug," affecting people in all socioeconomic groups and geographic areas of the U.S. It is much less expensive now—about 50% cheaper than a few years ago—and smoking cocaine ("freebasing"), a previously obscure underground practice, has become an extraordinarily widespread phenomenon since ready made freebase known as "crack" has appeared for sale on street corners in almost every urban area. While there is recent evidence suggesting that cocaine use has begun to decline in certain subgroups, the cocaine production and import trade continues to flourish, indeed to expand. We are forced to conclude either that those who are already addicted are using greater and greater quantities or that studies showing drops in cocaine use are not accurately reflecting use patterns. Furthermore, statistics on crack use indicate steady increases in availability and use.

IMPACT OF THE COCAINE OUTBREAK

The cocaine outbreak has had a reverberating impact throughout American society. In a very real sense, cocaine has been the "straw to break the camel's back" of the long-standing resistance to confronting illegal drug use in our society. Americans have been involved in a 25–30-year "love affair" with illegal drugs, evidenced by a continuous succession of changing drug trends since the '60s, with cocaine being only the latest development. The cocaine outbreak has heightened public consciousness and precipitated public outrage about the unacceptably high levels of drug abuse that persist among adolescents and adults. It has sparked public debates, anti-drug legislation, law enforcement efforts, and the establishment of drug prevention programs in schools. It has generated unprecedented concern about drug and alcohol use in the workplace, especially where public trust and safety are at stake. This has fostered implementation of employee urine testing procedures and an expansion of employee assistance programs aimed at identifying and treating substance abusers. The epidemic has even helped to make the prevention and treatment of illegal drug use a long-overdue national priority, as reflected by the level of importance it has assumed as a major issue in congressional and presidential elections and debates.

Nowhere has the impact of the cocaine epidemic been felt more dramatically than in the health care system, where the sharp escalation of cocaine use among the general public has led to a dramatic increase in the numbers of users seeking treatment. Health care systems are being strained by the recent explosion of cocaine use. Hospital emergency rooms, medical clinics, psychiatric clinics, and the private offices of physicians and psychotherapists all continue to be beseiged by people seeking help for cocaine-related problems. Most profoundly affected by the influx of cocaine users are drug abuse and alcoholism treatment programs and rehabilitation centers, most of which were established long before the recent cocaine outbreak.

Traditionally, drug abuse treatment programs were set up to deal with heroin addicts and alcoholism treatment programs to deal with alcoholics. No one anticipated the current epidemic and so the entire treatment system was literally caught off guard by the rapid influx of cocaine users. To the staff of these programs, cocaine addicts represent a new breed of patient whose demographics, personality profiles, and life experiences differ significantly from those who appeared for treatment in the past. This phenomenon has placed new, unanticipated demands on the existing treatment system to adapt or overhaul its strategies in order to meet the clinical needs of these patients. While there are probably more similarities than differences between various types of chemical addictions, the differences that do exist are often crucial to the outcome of treatment. For example, consider how vastly different the focus of initial treatment is likely to be with a heroin addict complaining of severe withdrawal symptoms, an alcoholic in the throes of mental confusion or delirium tremens, and the cocaine addict who has no physical discomfort but is riddled with cravings and urges for the drug. Of course, the differences go far beyond those stemming from pharmacological variables alone. People use drugs for different reasons and for different desired effects. One's choice of a particular drug is never purely an accident, especially with so many different drugs available to choose from.

The wave of cocaine users seeking treatment has already prompted significant changes in the addiction treatment field. At the most fundamental level it has forced a reevaluation of traditional definitions of addiction and addictive drugs. When cocaine users began to seek treatment because they could not stop using the drug despite the absence of withdrawal symptoms, experts were forced to look a little closer at the compulsive cravings and drug-seeking behavior propelled by a complex set of interrelated forces, from cellular biochemical changes in the brain to behavioral conditioning factors. Addiction could no longer be understood mainly in terms of avoiding physical withdrawal discomfort. This revised thinking has, in turn, given new legitimacy to nonchemical addictions, such as compulsive gambling, compulsive sexuality, compulsive spending, and compulsive eating — areas of human suffering that are just now attracting serious investigation.

The cocaine outbreak has forced the existing treatment system to better adapt itself to the clinical needs of the employed, middle-class drug user. This has placed a greater emphasis on shortening the length of stay in residential programs and increasing the utilization of intensive outpatient programs in order to avoid unnecessary disruption to the patient's work and home life and to contain skyrocketing treatment costs. There has been a proliferation of private, confidential, comfortable, professionally staffed treatment programs designed to better meet the demands of the middle-class substance abuser. Drug abuse treatment programs housed in dismal store-front locations have had to change their appearance and strategies in order to attract a somewhat more savvy and sophisticated clientele. The typical outpatient counseling center of the '60s and '70s had a high relapse rate among patients, probably because what we now know to be basic ingredients for effective treatment were lacking: Outpatient programs were nonintensive and loosely structured, in many cases offering only one counseling session per week and little or no group support; patients were rarely required to remain abstinent from alcohol and marijuana; families were only occasionally involved; neither staff nor patients were given education about addictive disease; the emphasis was on getting patients off their drug of choice rather than staying off; and participation of patients in self-help groups was rarely encouraged.

The cocaine outbreak has motivated health care providers from many different professional disciplines to become better educated about substance abuse disorders and their treatment. In the '60s and '70s, when illegal drug use was associated with rebellious teenagers smoking pot or dropping acid or with poor inner-city blacks and hispanics shooting heroin, drug abusers were viewed by health care professionals as being on the fringe of society, well outside the mainstream of medical and psychiatric care. When educated, middle-class business executives, corporate employees, and professionals began seeking treatment for cocaine addiction, attitudes about drug addiction began to change. Now that drug addicts are appearing throughout the health care system, clinicians from virtually all disciplines (especially those in the mental health professions) are recognizing the need to become better educated about the problem and its treatment. Unfortunately, few physicians or psychotherapists are experienced in the proper diagnosis and treat-

ment of addicted persons, but professional training programs and confer-
ences are at least trying to correct this deficiency.

The cocaine outbreak has helped to narrow the long-standing gap between professionals in the alcoholism and substance abuse treatment fields.
The days of the so-called "pure" drug addict or alcoholic are numbered.
Very few cocaine abusers are involved only with cocaine and very few alcohol abusers are involved only with alcohol. Cocaine abusers drink alcohol to
"come down" from the unpleasant stimulant effects of cocaine. Alcohol
abusers snort cocaine in order to "wake up" from the depressant effects of
alcohol. Drug abuse counselors are faced with having to better understand
alcoholism in order to deal effectively with drug abusers. Similarly, alcoholism counselors are faced with having to better understand cocaine and other
forms of drug abuse in order to deal effectively with alcoholics. Not only are
more chemical abusers combining different substances, but now alcohol is
recognized as a major factor promoting relapse to cocaine, just as cocaine is
recognized as a major factor promoting relapse to alcohol. Professional
training workshops on cocaine now routinely include discussions of relevant
alcohol issues, while workshops on alcohol include discussions of relevant
cocaine and other drug issues. As a result, interaction between these two
previously separate groups of professionals and the historically separate
government agencies that regulate alcoholism and drug abuse treatment has
begun to flourish.

Recognition of the importance of treating "the disease within" is a pivotal
development of recent years in the drug abuse treatment field, resulting in
part from the cocaine outbreak. There is now a discernible shift away from
helping patients to merely get off drugs and an increasing emphasis on
helping them to stay off over the long term. Stopping drug use is easy
enough in most cases, especially when there are no withdrawal symptoms to
contend with (as is true with cocaine): It's staying stopped (i.e., preventing
relapse) that is the key to long-term success. This shift has occurred in part
because of the increased demand for drug abuse treatment and the relative
failure of efforts that have focused almost exclusively on detoxification. In
fact, the lifelong vulnerability to relapse is now regarded as a standard
diagnostic feature of all chemical dependency problems, and the emerging
consensus is that the task of preventing relapse must be addressed directly
and specifically.

Expanding the definition of addiction, spurred largely by the cocaine
epidemic, has wrought yet another change: a trend in drug treatment toward
requiring total abstinence from all drugs, not just the patient's drug of
choice. In the 1960s and 1970s, many drug abuse treatment programs required patients to abstain completely from their drug of choice (usually
heroin), but ignored or permitted the use of alcohol, marijuana, and even

cocaine—since these drugs were perceived as being relatively benign and nonaddictive and use of them was not seen as contrary or damaging to the patient's treatment. The fact that drinking or use of other drugs could set off craving for the patient's drug of choice, reduce his/her ability to resist temptation, or lead to substitute addictions was not given adequate consideration. This lack of recognition of the dangers of any mood-altering chemical use as an important relapse factor, coupled with the lack of application of the disease model as the fundamental basis for treatment, probably contributed significantly to the notoriously low success rates in most treatment programs. The disease model states that once a person has crossed the line from chemical use to chemical addiction he/she can never return to controlled use without rekindling the addiction. Furthermore, this model holds not just for the person's drug of choice, but for all psychoactive or mood-altering substances, thus underscoring the need for total abstinence as the first and foremost treatment goal. While routinely used in treatment programs for alcoholics, the disease model has been historically absent from programs treating drug addicts. Clearly, growing acceptance of addiction as a disease is transforming the drug abuse treatment field in this particular area; as a result, relapse rates are decreasing.

The cocaine epidemic may be telling us that we are now more vulnerable to drug addiction—and all addictions—than ever before, that susceptibility to addictions is spreading in our culture. It isn't just media hype that prompts us repeatedly to watch TV specials, listen to radio programs, and read newspaper and magazine articles on cocaine and crack. No, we are riveted to our television sets and buying out the newsstands because the cocaine epidemic is showing us something quite scary: Drug addiction can happen to anyone; we are all vulnerable. Since there is no longer a single demographic profile of the typical cocaine user, clinicians must be prepared to treat a diverse group of patients: blue collar, white collar, unemployed, suburban, inner-city, male, female, middle-aged, adolescent, cross-addicted, and those with or without psychiatric disorders. Some people question whether the cocaine epidemic, like any other illness whose incidence increases when immunity is weakened, is exposing something fundamentally wrong with the American mentality, culture, or way of life. Such basic questions remain to be answered in the coming decades; at least the phenomenon of cocaine addiction among the middle class has led us to begin asking these questions in the first place.

Treating drug abusers has never been considered an easy task. The high staff "burnout" rate observed in the drug treatment field has stood as evidence that this area of specialty was ideal only for those willing to work long hours with few rewards. The fact is that, with an informed treatment approach and a reasonably motivated patient, the prognosis for recovery from substance abuse, including cocaine addiction, may actually be better than that for most other mental health problems. Success rates will depend, of course, on a variety of factors, including the severity of addiction, the patient's motivation to recover, and the extent to which the program provides critical treatment ingredients, such as those described in this book. The best prognosis exists for those patients with a strong desire to stop using cocaine, social supports to do so, a history of good functioning before cocaine addiction, and a willingness to accept the need for lifestyle change and total abstinence. The fact that success rates can be good was shown in a study of 127 cocaine addicts who entered my outpatient treatment program. Over 65 percent completed the six-to-twelve-month program and over 75 percent of these patients were still drug-free at one-to-two-year follow-up.

PURPOSE OF THIS BOOK

The purpose of this book is to provide any interested reader with a step-by-step description of effective treatment for cocaine addiction. For the person who is addicted to cocaine or concerned about someone with the problem, this book can serve as an informative guide to the treatment process. It:

- provides basic information about cocaine and cocaine addiction;
- describes the disease model of cocaine addiction, including an explanation of how this model enhances the treatment and recovery process;
- describes cocaine's effects on the human brain in easily understood terms in order to enhance the reader's appreciation for the biological factors in cocaine addiction;
- defines the criteria for deciding when a cocaine addict requires hospitalization or can be treated successfully as an outpatient;
- discusses specific techniques for preventing relapse to cocaine;
- describes the complementary roles of self-help and professional treatment and how to maximize the benefits of each;
- describes the impact of cocaine addiction on the family and how family members can be of help in the treatment process;
- describes what a good treatment program should consist of and how it should work, making the difficult task of finding a good program more than just a shot in the dark.

For the clinician with or without prior experience in treating cocaine abusers, it provides a highly practical, detailed guide to the clinical assessment and treatment of cocaine addicts on an outpatient basis. The major purpose of the book is to help the reader funnel clinical knowledge and experience into a model of treatment that works. It takes the reader through the successive steps of assessment, treatment planning, establishing initial abstinence, preventing relapse, and laying the foundation for long-term recovery. Assessment forms and patient hand-outs are provided to facilitate the practical application of suggested treatment techniques. It describes the fundamental differences between treating alcoholics and cocaine addicts. Techniques of group therapy, individual therapy, and family therapy are discussed as well as techniques of treatment contracting, urine testing, and managing relapses. The special topics of treating cocaine-addicted adolescents, women, athletes, and health-care professionals are also covered.

Most of the clinical material in this book is based on my own experience in treating hundreds, if not thousands, of cocaine addicts and in developing treatment programs aimed at being maximally effective with these patients. The emphasis of this book is on outpatient treatment and specific techniques that appear to work best in that treatment setting. This reflects not only the increasing emphasis of my clinical work in recent years, but also a growing nationwide trend stimulated by a combination of clinical and economic considerations. Outpatient as compared to inpatient (residential) treatment is more acceptable to the majority of cocaine addicts and less expensive to the patient, to government funding agencies, and to third-party payers such as health insurance companies. With the proliferation of outpatient programs, more treatment can be provided with fewer dollars, thus making much-needed help accessible to larger numbers of people.

Those suffering from cocaine addiction cannot wait for scientific studies to identify the most effective treatment approaches—they need help right now. What we already know about the treatment of this problem is more than adequate to offer the hope of successful recovery to many, if not most. Furthermore, it is highly unlikely that any single treatment method will prove to be best for all cocaine addicts. The key to successful treatment is individualized treatment planning which provides a good match between the patient's clinical needs and the treatment strategies employed to meet those needs. The starting point of all good treatment is a thorough, sensitive, sophisticated assessment of the nature and severity of the patient's problem—a topic covered extensively in this book.

This book does not profess to offer the final word on the treatment of cocaine addiction. It is intended to convey to the reader practical, useful information based on direct clinical experience. Toward this goal, I have not hesitated to convey my clinical impressions, opinions, and suggestions in the absence of scientific validation. In the years to follow, there will no doubt be new developments that expand, refine, modify, or replace many of the techniques described here. For now, if this book makes effective treatment of cocaine addiction more understandable and more available to even a few who suffer from the problem, it will have succeeded in its intended goal.

CHAPTER 1

Cocaine: What You Need to Know

IN ORDER TO TREAT cocaine addicts successfully, thorough knowledge and understanding of the particulars of cocaine use are essential. Treatment professionals who want to be effective with cocaine addicts must acquire a solid working knowledge of the basic issues, including the unique pharmacology of cocaine; its positive and negative effects; the different methods and routes of administration; the pharmacological, psychological, and cultural factors that drive people toward compulsive patterns of use; and the rituals associated with purchasing, preparing, and using cocaine in its many and varied forms.

Every drug has its own ethos, folklore, and special appeal to a subgroup of users. The patient's choice of drug is neither random nor inconsequential. Although there may be many similarities among addicts who choose one mood-altering substance as opposed to another, the differences are noteworthy as well. Cocaine addicts are not merely alcoholics or heroin addicts who have accidentally chosen a different drug. This is an important point and one to keep in mind throughout this book as we attempt to better understand the specifics of cocaine addiction and its treatment.

The cocaine addict who comes for treatment wants assurance that the professional who is offering help knows what he/she is talking about when it comes to drugs and drug use. The prospective patient will not feel sufficiently confident and secure if the professional's knowledge about drug use is

10

merely superficial. The clinician must be able to inform and educate the patient, rather than vice versa.

THE BASICS

Cocaine Hydrochloride Powder

Most cocaine available in the United States is imported and sold in the form of cocaine hydrochloride powder. This is a white, odorless, crystalline substance, derived from the leaves of the coca plant, *Erythroxylon coca*, grown primarily in the mountainous regions of Central and South America.

Cocaine powder is sold on the illicit street market at prices ranging from $75 to $100 per gram with purities ranging from approximately 30 to 75 percent. Nearly 100 percent pure pharmaceutical cocaine, diverted from legal suppliers, has been available at times on the illicit market, but tighter controls in recent years have drastically reduced the supply. Those using pharmaceutical cocaine are likely to be health professionals who self-prescribe or divert hospital supplies.

Cocaine hydrochloride is legally classified by the U.S. Food and Drug Administration as a Schedule II drug (high abuse potential with limited medical usefulness). It is still used sometimes as a local anesthetic in nasal and eye surgery.

Pharmacologic Actions

Cocaine has two main pharmacologic actions. It is both a local anesthetic and a central nervous system (CNS) stimulant—the only drug known to possess both of these properties.

Cocaine exerts its local anesthetic (numbing or "freezing") actions, similar to novocaine or xylocaine used routinely in dental procedures, by blocking the conduction of sensory impulses within nerve cells. This effect is most pronounced when the drug is applied to the skin or to mucous membranes. Cocaine hydrochloride has long been used legitimately as a local anesthetic in surgery of the nose, throat, and larynx. Because of its local anesthetic actions, when cocaine is "snorted" it temporarily numbs the user's nasal and throat passages—an effect known to all experienced users. Dealers looking to increase their profits often capitalize on this by adding cheaper local anesthetics such as procaine, lidocaine, or tetracaine to their cocaine in order to reduce its purity (and thus raise profits), while retaining the drug's anticipated effects.

Cocaine's CNS stimulant effects are mediated primarily by its effects on

neurotransmitters (chemical messengers) in the brain, such as norepinephrine and dopamine. The exact mechanism by which cocaine exerts these
effects is uncertain, but it is thought that cocaine both increases the release
of these neurotransmitters at nerve cell endings (synapses) and prolongs
their actions. It also stimulates sympathetic activity in the peripheral nervous system, which gives rise to increased heart rate, blood pressure, breathing rate, body temperature, blood sugar, and dilation of the pupils. In
combination with its direct stimulant effect on the brain, these changes give
the user a strong feeling of being more alert and energetic.

These responses are very similar to the body's normal physiological response to threat, the primitive survival mechanism known as the "fight or
flight" response. Its similarity to this natural emergency reaction or warning
system may explain cocaine's tendency to cause exaggerated feelings of anxiety and paranoia at higher doses.

Another one of cocaine's stimulant effects is vasoconstriction, narrowing
of the blood vessels, an action that helps to prolong the drug's local anesthetic action by preventing it from being absorbed too quickly into the
surrounding circulation. The vasoconstrictive effect has sometimes been
utilized in medicine to help limit bleeding during delicate surgery of the nose
and eyes.

Although cocaine is now classified as a Schedule II controlled substance,
it has been erroneously classified for many years as a narcotic along with
heroin, opium, morphine, and other opiates. While it is correct to categorize
cocaine as a dangerous addictive substance, calling it a narcotic is technical-
ly inaccurate. The word "narcotic" derives from the Greek "narkotikos,"
which means "sleep-inducing." Opiates such as heroin *are* narcotics in that
they depress the central nervous system, decreasing alertness and interest in
the immediate environment. Cocaine, a potent stimulant drug, has exactly
the opposite effects.

METHODS OF USE

Three methods of self-administering cocaine are common in the United
States today: snorting, smoking, and intravenous (IV) injection.

Snorting Cocaine

Intranasal use or sniffing it up the nostrils — called "snorting" — is by far
the most popular method of using cocaine, partly because of the erroneous
yet persistent belief that when used in this way cocaine is relatively nonaddictive and harmless. Many people still believe the myth that intranasal use

is self-limiting, although it is now clear that many cocaine snorters become addicted.

Cocaine snorters typically prepare the drug for use by placing it on a smooth flat surface (such as a mirror, piece of glass, or marble), chop the crystalline substance into a fine powdery consistency with a razor blade, and push it into very narrow lines, one or two inches in length. A straw or rolled-up dollar bill is then used to sniff it up into the nostrils. Or, a small amount of cocaine is taken onto a tiny "coke spoon," which is then lifted up to the opening of the nostril to be inhaled.

Once inhaled, cocaine is absorbed into the small blood vessels of the mucous membrane lining the nose. From there it travels through the general venous system to the vena cava, to the right heart, out into the blood vessels of the lungs, to the left heart, and from there to the brain. It takes about five minutes or so after snorting cocaine until the user starts to feel the high. The concentration of cocaine in the blood peaks between 15 minutes and one hour after ingestion, while the high itself may last for 20–30 minutes.

"Just snorting" cocaine does not provide immunity from addiction; it simply takes longer for addiction to occur with this method of use than by injecting or smoking cocaine. Over a long enough period of time and in sufficient doses, intranasal use does cause addiction; in fact, the majority of those who become dependent on cocaine are primarily intranasal users. While proportionately fewer intranasal users probably end up addicted as compared to IV users or freebase smokers, the majority of cocaine addicts are snorters.

The preparatory ritual involved in sniffing cocaine, as with that for injecting or smoking cocaine, appears to play some part in the addiction conditioning process as well. A recovering cocaine addict who so much as sees cocaine paraphernalia or a pile of cocaine on TV or in a magazine may experience intense cravings and urges for the drug, particularly if this happens in the early stages of cocaine abstinence.

Some cocaine users seek status images of affluence and glamour for themselves, as reflected in the high-currency bills, gold-plated straws, or coke spoons incorporated into their drug-use rituals. Ironically, of course, users who become dependent on the drug commonly lose any affluence they might have had to begin with, and when beset with such problems as severe weight loss, paranoia, and depression those under chemical control of cocaine would be hard-pressed to appear glamorous.

Due to the irritating chemicals in cocaine and its additives, snorting cocaine on a regular basis can cause ulcerations (sores) in the mucous membrane lining the nose. It can also cause nosebleeds and in some cases perforation of the nasal septum — a hole in the cartilage separating the nostrils.

Smoking Cocaine

Some users prefer to smoke rather than snort cocaine. To smoke cocaine, the cocaine powder must first be converted into a smokeable form known as "freebase" or "crack." This is easily done by means of a simple chemical conversion procedure utilizing baking soda, water, and heat. Until several years ago, ether rather than baking soda was used routinely as the solvent or reagent to make freebase, but its explosive quality, brought to public attention by the severe burns suffered by Richard Pryor (a self-admitted cocaine freebase addict), has led to its replacement by baking soda (sodium bicarbonate) — a non-explosive chemical that is much cheaper and more accessible than ether.

Cocaine powder cannot be efficiently smoked because it decomposes when heated; that is, most of the active drug is destroyed at temperatures achieved by a regular match or lighter. Thus, the user who attempts to smoke cocaine powder derives little if any psychoactive effects ("high") from the drug. To convert cocaine powder into a form that can be smoked, the *basic* cocaine alkaloid must be chemically *freed* from its hydrochloride salt — thus the name "freebase" for the end product of this process.

Perhaps because cigarette smoking is so common in our society and because marijuana has often been regarded as less dangerous than other illicit drugs, many people assume that smoking a drug is not as harmful as injecting one. In fact, smoking a drug delivers higher doses of it into the brain more quickly than any other route of administration — even IV use. When taken directly into the lungs, cocaine immediately enters the pulmonary circulation (the peripheral venous system is bypassed) and reaches the brain in only 8–10 seconds.

As mentioned earlier, crack and freebase are the same drug. But there is still much confusion about the terminology. The noun "freebase" refers to the cocaine base or alkaloid that is chemically released or freed from its hydrochloride salt so that it can be volatized into smoke without decomposing. Similarly the verb "freebasing" refers to the process of *smoking* freebase — not to the process of *making* freebase. Crack users rarely if ever use the word "freebase" to describe their drug use. They simply say that they smoke crack. For clinical purposes, however, there is absolutely no difference between smoking crack and smoking freebase.

Although crack is readily available on the streets, many freebasers continue to buy the powder and make their own freebase. The preparation procedure itself has become a part of their drug use ritual. An informal status system has now developed among cocaine users, with crack smokers being regarded as lower in status (many are from lower socioeconomic groups), while freebase smokers somehow retain a degree of snob appeal as more middle-class users. Both crack and self-converted freebase are usually smoked by crumbling the substance into the small bowl of a special glass water pipe. In the pipe the smoke passes through a bulb that is filled with water to cool the hot vapors. The user ignites the drug and inhales the smoke deeply, retaining it in the lungs as long as possible, to maximize absorption, as marijuana smokers do.

The high from smoking freebase or crack is short-lived, lasting two to five minutes, after which the user's mood drops rapidly. The crash from freebase or crack is proportionately as intense as the high, and sets in abruptly, as soon as the brief high wears off. The symptoms of the crash are the same as with snorting—irritability, depression, and anxiety accompanied by drug cravings—but more severe.

Many freebase smokers are unaware of the fact that the process of converting cocaine powder to freebase does not remove most of the contaminants or "cuts" typically found in cocaine powder bought on the street. Neither self-prepared freebase nor crack is "pure." Many of the active "cuts" survive the extraction process and are delivered into the bloodstream and brain in more concentrated doses—making them more dangerous and more likely to cause a toxic reaction.

The appearance of crack on the illicit drug market has dramatically increased the number of people who smoke freebase. By making the highly addictive, smokeable form of cocaine readily available with "no fuss, no muss," at an introductory trial price affordable to almost anyone, dealers have expanded their market astronomically in a short period of time. Crack is like a "fast-food" version of cocaine—it's preprepared, cheap, readily available, doesn't last long, and leaves the user wanting more.

Since the introduction of crack, particular segments of the cocaine-using population appear to have been tapped, namely lower-income people and teenagers. These subgroups may have previously found cocaine to be out of their reach financially, but with crack they have found it not only affordable but readily available.

Crack is not cheap, however. It only seems cheap because it is sold in such small quantities. On a weight-for-weight basis, it is actually twice as expensive as cocaine powder. Not only that, but addiction to crack occurs so fast that the user often buys greater and greater quantities more and more often, resulting in a very expensive crack habit indeed. Many crack addicts report spending hundreds of dollars a day for the drug—hardly an inexpensive bargain!

Because of the more intense crash and concomitant cravings for more cocaine, freebase and crack smokers often chain smoke until their supply is gone. This type of marathon binge use, which may last for hours or even days, is called a "run." Freebase smokers may use ten times as much cocaine as intranasal users in a given time period, primarily because of this binge use. A "run" can cost a freebaser hundreds or even thousands of dollars a day, and leave him/her in a state of total dysfunction.

It follows that freebase and crack smokers, in addition to becoming addicted rapidly, often display more severe psychiatric symptoms, such as paranoia, severe depression, and emotional volatility. Consequently they are capable of erupting into violent, suicidal, or homicidal acts. Also, because of the large, concentrated doses that reach the brain, seizures are more likely to occur from smoking cocaine than from snorting it, and smoking can lead more easily to respiratory failure and/or cardiac arrest. Heart attacks and strokes are also more common: blood pressure can increase dramatically with cocaine's vasoconstrictive effects, raising the risk of restricting blood flow to the heart or brain tissue. Increased heart rate or erratic heart rhythms may worsen existing heart conditions, including those of which the user may not even be aware.

Further, holding in the hot vapors for long periods of time can severely irritate the lungs, resulting in wheezing, chest congestion, and coughing up black phlegm. When the lungs are irritated from smoking cocaine, there is a greater vulnerability to bronchial infections, pneumonia, and other respiratory problems. Cocaine smokers may also risk serious lung damage. According to recent studies, lung cells may be damaged by repeated exposure to both the cocaine and its "cuts," limiting diffusing capacity, the lung's life-sustaining ability to exchange oxygen and carbon dioxide from the bloodstream. Such damage shows up as shortness of breath and a constant cough. It is not yet known whether or not this damage is fully reversible.

Because addiction brought on by smoking cocaine is often quite severe, cravings and the resulting propensity to relapse are also more likely. Successful recovery is also made proportionately more difficult.

Injecting Cocaine

Finally, since cocaine powder is soluble in water, a solution of the drug can be drawn up in a syringe for injection, sometimes mixed in the same syringe with heroin — a drug combination known as a "speedball." The appeal of this drug "cocktail" stems from the ability of heroin to dampen the unpleasant jitteriness and crash from cocaine, yielding a calmer drug-induced euphoria. Some speedball users, however, get "calmer" than they bargained for. The speedball is particularly dangerous for a few reasons. First, heroin lowers respiration rate, and in high enough doses cocaine does too. Together, the two drugs may halt respiration completely. Second, opiates lower the threshold for brain seizures. Because cocaine is capable of inducing brain seizures by itself, combining it with heroin makes the occurrence of a seizure all the more likely. Third, misinformation surrounding the speedball poses a special danger. Users may think that combining the two drugs is actually safer than using either drug alone, under the assumption that they "cancel each other out." In believing so, they may use at least their usual amount of each, adding up to a whopping total chemical dose. The result: 66 percent of cocaine-related deaths in a recent coroner's report were attributed to speedball combinations.

Relatively few intravenous (IV) cocaine users start or switch to IV administration without a prior history of IV heroin use. The popularity of IV cocaine use may be on the decline because of rising concern about contracting AIDS and also because the intense "rush" of cocaine euphoria produced by IV administration can be achieved just as readily by smoking cocaine freebase, without any risk of infection from contaminated needles. IV drug users have always run the risk of contracting serious diseases (such as hepatitis) by sharing "dirty" (used) hypodermic needles. Now, of course, there is the additional, critical danger of contracting AIDS, transmitted through the blood. IV users, in the grips of a craving or withdrawal syndrome, rarely concern themselves with *any* long-range ramifications of their behavior, instead seeking relief from their immediate distress. So, given the reality of compulsive drug use, the very nature of drug addiction, any IV user today is in extreme danger.

The intravenous user begins his/her ritual of drug preparation by placing roughly one-eighth or one-quarter of a gram of cocaine on a spoon, adding a little bit of water and dissolving the cocaine to form the aqueous solution, and then straining it through a tiny, mesh strainer. The solution is finally drawn up into a syringe and injected directly into a vein.

From the vein into which it is injected, the cocaine travels back to the right side of the heart, out to the lungs, to the left side of the heart, and up to the brain, completing its journey in about 30–60 seconds. The high occurs almost as quickly as with smoking cocaine, and with similar intensity. The high also wears off quickly and in most cases is followed by an equally intense crash. Blood levels of cocaine peak about five minutes after IV injection.

Similar to freebase smoking, this roller-coaster action promotes repeated injections, as the user seeks to escape the crash, obtain the euphoria again, and satisfy the cravings caused by dopamine depletion in the brain. Thus, users often engage in binge use, marathon "runs" of nearly continuous use lasting hours or even days, during which extraordinarily high doses are consumed. The risk of addiction and of psychiatric and medical consequences is as high for IV users as it is for freebase smokers, if not higher.

Buying Cocaine and Crack on the Street

Cocaine powder is usually bought in units of a gram — approximately two heaping teaspoonfuls — at street prices ranging from $75 to $100. A gram of cocaine will yield roughly 10–15 "lines." These are individual doses of the drug arranged in straight lines two or three inches long on a flat surface. Each line is taken into the nostril, usually in a single prolonged and forceful inhalation delivering anywhere from 10 to 20 milligrams of cocaine, depending on the purity of the supply.

A gram of cocaine may not last very long for a heavy user, especially not for freebase smokers or IV users who tend to consume large quantities in short periods of time in the course of marathon binges. Thus, heavy users often buy cocaine in quantities larger than a gram in order to have enough of the drug to meet their own consumption levels. Also, cocaine is cheaper when purchased in larger quantities. For example, some users buy the drug in ounces rather than grams. An ounce is approximately 28 grams. If an ounce of cocaine is bought for $1,400 (a typical price), the buyer is paying only $50 a gram — a substantial bargain compared to the price of $75 to $100 per gram when purchased in smaller amounts. Similarly, to get a substantial but somewhat smaller price break, cocaine can be purchased by the "quarter" (a quarter ounce or 7 grams) or by the "eighth" (an eighth of an ounce or 3.5 grams).

The process of buying "crack" rather than cocaine powder is entirely different. Unlike freebasers who first buy the cocaine powder and then convert it themselves into smokeable freebase, "crack" users buy the already preprepared freebase (ready to smoke with no further processing) directly from the dealer and thus need not perform the chemical conversion process. Again, "crack" and freebase are the same drug; the different names connote only who performed the extraction process: the dealer (in the case of crack) or the buyer (in the case of freebase).

Unlike cocaine powder, "crack" is not sold by the gram or ounce. It is sold by the "rock" — small pea-size beige pellets of freebase dispensed in tiny plastic vials (see Figure 1.1). A crack vial may sell for $5 to $35 dollars, depending on the number and size of the "rocks" inside it. Smoking cocaine can become a very expensive habit very quickly. One rock typically yields only four or five "hits" (inhalations) of cocaine vapors. The effects of each hit may last only four or five minutes before the desire for more cocaine sets in. Freebase or crack is almost always smoked in a glass waterpipe (or sometimes a makeshift "pipe" constructed from a soda can) using a butane lighter or "torch" as the heat source. Some users smoke it mixed with tobacco and/or marijuana in a cigarette, but with this less efficient method of drug delivery the effects are not as intense and more of the drug is wasted.

FIGURE 1.1

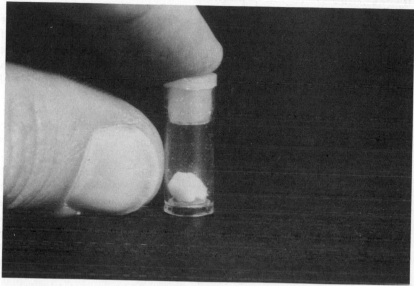

Courtesy of U.S. Drug Enforcement Agency, New York Field Division.

Cocaine "Cuts"

To increase profits, all street dealers mix or "cut" cocaine with other substances to increase its volume and weight. This means that buyers never know for sure exactly what they are buying and, more importantly, what they are actually putting into their body and brain. Generally, two types of cuts or adulterants are used: (1) active cuts — those which mimic specific pharmacologic effects of cocaine — and (2) inactive cuts — those which usually have no pharmacologic actions but are similar in appearance to cocaine.

Active cuts. These are substitute drugs with distinct physiological and/or mood-altering actions of their own that are used as adulterants to actively mimic one or more effects of cocaine. For example, local anesthetic drugs, such as procaine and lidocaine, are commonly used because like cocaine they numb any tissue or membrane that they touch. The dealer than touts the mixture as "good stuff," and if the customer puts it on his lips or tongue or snorts a line, the expected numbing effects are all there.

CNS stimulants (including amphetamines) are also commonly used as active cuts to mimic the rapid heartbeat and flushed, energized feeling induced by cocaine. The user who tries this mix may be readily convinced that it's a "good buy," even though a substantial portion of the effects may be from the adulterants and not from cocaine.

Inactive cuts. These are filler substances that are largely devoid of any psychoactive or physiological effects of their own and are added simply to dilute the cocaine by increasing its volume and weight. These substances usually resemble cocaine powder in appearance and texture. Common inert cuts include mannitol (a relatively safe commercial filler used in the manufacture of various pills), lactose and dextrose powders (sugars), and inositol (a B vitamin). Other inactive cuts include cornstarch, flour, and talcum powder.

"SPACEBASING"

A small number of users report smoking crack that has been sprinkled with liquid PCP, or phencyclidine (also known as "angel dust"). This practice, called "spacebasing," produces a powerful combination of stimulant, anesthetic, and hallucinogenic effects. It is capable of prompting intense feelings of panic, terror, and in some cases unpredictable, violent, uncontrollable behavior. Because smoking crack can itself produce intense paranoid and violent behavior, its combination with PCP is particularly dangerous. Spacebasing does not appear widespread at this time, but has appeared intermittently but infrequently in the New York City and Los Angeles areas.

If at all possible, a user under the influence of this combination should be treated where restraint can safely be applied, as in a hospital emergency room or psychiatric unit. Under all other conditions, treatment professionals should proceed with extreme caution, seeking only to calm the patient, removing all extraneous stimuli, and avoiding any action that could be construed by the patient as threatening.

COCA PASTE—"BASUCO"

Another smokeable form of cocaine, perhaps the most dangerous, is coca paste or "basuco." This crude product is made in South America by using gasoline, kerosene, and sulfuric acid to extract a pasty smokeable substance from the coca plant leaves. The paste is then dried and smoked in a pipe or crumbled into a cigarette, much like crack or freebase.

Because of its high concentration and rapid delivery to the brain, coca paste can cause rapid addiction and severe medical and psychiatric dysfunction. In addition, traces of kerosene and leaded gasoline remain in the paste and when smoked can cause severe irreversible lung damage as well as lead poisoning of liver and brain. This highly toxic form of cocaine has been distributed primarily in cocaine-producing countries of South America, where many users have suffered severe consequences. Drug enforcement agencies in the United States report that with the exception of several isolated reports, which have not been substantiated, coca paste is not available here—yet.

CHAPTER 2

Why Do People Use Cocaine?

PEOPLE TAKE COCAINE mainly to alter their brain function and thereby alter their mood and mental state. The acute positive effects of cocaine (the "high") are all a direct result of cocaine-induced biochemical changes in brain activity, which produce desired changes in mood and consciousness. As with all mood-altering drugs, the state of cocaine intoxication is difficult to describe. Moreover, both the quality and intensity of the cocaine-induced experience can vary markedly according to many different factors, including: the dosage; the chronicity of use; the method of drug administration; the simultaneous use of other drugs; the mood, personality, expectations, and physical condition of the user; the reasons for taking the drug; and the setting and circumstances under which the drug is taken. Not all users get the same effects. Even within the same person, the effects can change drastically with increasing dosages and chronicity of use. The cocaine "high" can change from extremely pleasant to extremely unpleasant and even terrifying as usage becomes more chronic and intensified.

COCAINE EFFECTS

Positive Mood-altering Effects

The acute positive effects of cocaine usually include a generalized state of euphoria in combination with feelings of increased energy, confidence, mental alertness, and sexual arousal. Many people feel more talkative, more intensely involved in their interaction with others, and more playful and spontaneous when high on cocaine. Preexisting shyness, tension, and fatigue may instantly disappear. Although in the early "honeymoon" stage of cocaine, positive effects predominate and few (if any) negative effects are present, some users do experience temporary unpleasant reactions and aftereffects. These may include feelings of restlessness, anxiety, agitation, irritability, and insomnia. Suspiciousness, confusion, hyperarousal, and elements of paranoid thinking may also appear even in nonchronic low-dose users, depending on the individual's susceptibility to these effects.

Negative Mood-altering Effects

With continued escalating use, the user becomes progressively tolerant to the positive effects while the negative effects steadily intensify. But the addicted individual persists in compulsive cocaine taking. The highs are not so high anymore and the rebound aftereffects return the user not to his/her former pre-cocaine involvement condition, but rather to an increasingly dysphoric, depressed state. This only re-initiates the desire for more cocaine in a futile attempt at mood normalization. What began as a search for the ultimate euphoric high leaves the user in the depths of depression and despair.

FACTORS THAT PROMOTE COMPULSIVE COCAINE USE

The "Pharmacologic Imperative" of Cocaine

The late Dr. Sidney Cohen, for many years a highly respected leader in the substance abuse treatment field, described what he termed the "pharmacologic imperative" of cocaine. As a long-term observer of the drug scene over several decades, Dr. Cohen was convinced that the powerfully rewarding properties of cocaine were capable of making obsessive users of even the most mature and well-integrated persons among us. A sinister chemist, he said, who wanted to design a drug that would purposefully entrap many users into addiction would have trouble designing one better than cocaine.

Let's take a look at some of the "pharmacologic imperatives" that contribute to the development of compulsive use.

BRAIN REINFORCEMENT

Animals will work incessantly — to the point of exhaustion, debilitation, or death — pressing a bar over 12,000 times for a single dose of cocaine. They will choose cocaine over food, water, sex, and life itself. They will endure extremely painful electric shocks, starvation, and ultimately die from self-administering fatal doses. As explained more fully in Chapter 3, cocaine has "radar" for brain reward circuits and is able to stimulate these pleasure centers in a way that overrides even the most basic survival-oriented behaviors. What cocaine-addicted animals demonstrate dramatically is that a self-destructive compulsion to take cocaine can indeed occur in the absence of personality disorders, depression, anxiety, situational stressors, or family dysfunction. When attempting to explain the behavior of cocaine-addicted animals, it's hard to invoke explanations based on psychopathology, developmental history, or "addictive personalities." Animal experiments uniquely demonstrate that the "raw" addiction potential of cocaine is extraordinary.

INTENSE BUT SHORT-LIVED EUPHORIA

The cocaine high is intensely pleasurable but very brief. Its brevity necessitates frequent refills to constantly recapture the fleeting sensation. Taking repeated doses spaced at shorter and shorter intervals is required in order to maintain the desired effects.

REBOUND DYSPHORIA—THE "CRASH"

There is a negative counterpart to cocaine-induced euphoria. As soon as the brief high wears off and cocaine levels in the blood begin to fall, the intensely pleasurable state is replaced by an equally unpleasurable one, called the "crash." It's like an immediate rebound withdrawal reaction that intensifies with dosage and chronicity of use. This rapid shift from ecstasy to misery within a matter of minutes or seconds can be a potent motivator to take another dose in order to return as quickly as possible to the desired state. The "crashing" cocaine user knows all too well that relief is only moments away—as long as more supplies of cocaine are within reach. Another dose quickly eliminates the dysphoria and restores the euphoria, at least for a few minutes. When cocaine supplies run out and no more is accessible, the unpleasant "crash" still demands relief. Thus, alcohol, sedatives, tranquilizers, or even heroin enter the picture as antidotes for the unpleasant cocaine aftereffects. When polydrug abuse is added to cocaine addiction, everything becomes worse.

TOLERANCE

With continued, intensified use a larger and larger dose of cocaine is required to achieve the same effect. Chronic users will self-administer doses that at an earlier stage of use would have been lethal. Especially during prolonged binges, successive doses produce decreasing euphoria and decreasing autonomic changes (heartbeat, blood pressure, etc), indicating the development of tolerance. In all chronic users, a point is reached where the drug no longer produces any pleasurable sensations at all—only unpleasant ones—but the compulsion to recapture the vividly remembered, illusive high propels a continuing futile chase for paradise lost.

Contrary to common sense, the compulsion to continue using cocaine persists despite the absence of pleasurable effects, in part because of the intense conditioning and in part because the intensifying dysphoria and chronic depression cry out for relief. Additionally, chronic users reach a point where their reward circuits become tolerant to all pleasurable stimulation, even refractory to it—whether drug-induced or not. At that point, nothing is rewarding: neither cocaine nor any of life's ordinary pleasures. In an effort to get out of this intolerable bind, the chronic user is likely to take more cocaine, but again with little or no positive effect—only momentary improvement from a state of depression and despair to a state of slightly less depression and despair. When the user reaches this point, the cocaine addiction trap has already been sprung.

PHYSICAL DEPENDENCE

Although it produces no dramatic withdrawal syndrome, cocaine is still physically addictive. The physical addiction to cocaine takes the form of potent urges and cravings for the drug resulting from chronic biochemical alteration in brain chemistry (see Chapter 3 for details). In addition, repeated exposure of brain cells to high concentrations of cocaine alters cellular metabolism in a way that produces distortions in thinking, reasoning, perceptions, and emotions—all of which serve to further perpetuate the irrational cycle of compulsive drug use.

RAPID DELIVERY TO THE BRAIN

The physical properties of cocaine allow the application of rapid delivery systems to improve the speed and efficiency of drug absorption into the blood and brain. When cocaine is smoked or taken IV, all of the pharmacologic imperatives that drive compulsive use are intensified; i.e., the addiction potential of cocaine becomes much greater. Cerebral penetration of cocaine and its impact on brain function are greater with the pulmonary (smoking) and intravenous routes. As compared to the high from snorting, the high produced by smoking cocaine is experienced more rapidly, more intensely, but more briefly. The "crash" is also intensified (the higher the high, the lower the crash). Tolerance and physical dependence develop more quickly. Thus, all of the factors which promote the cocaine compulsion are accelerated and exaggerated when the rapid delivery systems of smoking or injecting are employed.

The Psychological and Cultural Imperatives of Cocaine

In addition to the pharmacologic properties of cocaine, there are at least several important psychological and cultural factors that contribute to compulsive cocaine use.

PSYCHIATRIC VULNERABILITY TO COCAINE

Inevitably, people who are unhappy, unstable, and psychiatrically disturbed as well as those with certain personality disorders, will probably always be overrepresented among substance abusers. Individuals in any type of compromised, negative mental state (whether temporary or permanent) are likely to find the offer of immediate chemical relief by cocaine and other drugs malignantly compelling and attractive. Narcissistic and borderline personality disorders are fairly prevalent in our general population and are even more so among those who seek all types of mental health services. It is no surprise, therefore, that people with these disorders are fairly common among the subpopulation of cocaine addicts as well. The unique ability of cocaine to instill feelings of self-confidence and self-control while simultaneously eliminating feelings of boredom and emptiness makes this drug especially appealing to those with narcissistic disturbances, i.e., to those who compensate for low self-esteem with exaggerated defenses of grandiosity, omnipotence, inflated self-importance, manipulative-exploitive use of others, and a facade of being in control and supremely self-sufficient. Interestingly, cocaine at first bolsters these narcissistic defenses, but eventually injures and incapacitates them as drug-related loss of control and dysfunction set in.

However, all such disturbed individuals will probably remain a distinct but significant *minority* of all substance abusers. As the use of certain mood-altering chemicals has become more normative in our society, psychopathology has become less important as either a necessary or sufficient precondition for becoming addicted. This is especially true under the current conditions, where cocaine and other drugs have never been more available, more potent, and more socially encouraged. Two additional points must be considered: (1) What is often referred to as psychopathology can be considered an adaptation to the experience of being a user of illegal drugs in a society which legally sanctions such behavior; and (2) psychiatric symptoms and aberrant behavior can be secondary to the drug use and a direct result of the biochemical and neurological insult to the brain caused by cocaine.

Many cocaine addicts who seek treatment do not exhibit any past or present psychiatric disturbance to speak of. It is difficult to agree with statements that most cocaine addicts suffer from preexisting dysthymia, hypomania, anxiety disorders, sociopathic personalities, etc. Exceptions abound. Further, such preconceptions often hinder rather than help the diagnostic and treatment process, since it is infinitely more effective to approach the cocaine addict as an addict rather than as a psychopath.

ADULT CHILDREN OF ALCOHOLICS/ADDICTS (ACOAS)

There is mounting evidence that the offspring of alcoholic parents are more likely to grow up and become alcoholic themselves, even if raised in a home with non-alcoholic foster parents. Probably both genetic and environ-ment/psychological factors are at work here. The vulnerability not only to alcoholism but also to cocaine addiction appears to be greater among people who come from families with alcohol or drug problems. In a cohort of 161 primary cocaine addicts who entered my outpatient treatment program, nearly half (41%) reported a history of severe alcohol or drug problems in parents and/or grandparents. Others working with cocaine addicts have noted equally high or higher rates of addiction in family members.

What appears to be transmitted from one generation to the next (biologi-cally and/or psychologically) is probably a nonspecific vulnerability to chemical dependency rather than an alcohol-specific or cocaine-specific pre-disposition. However, because of its higher addiction potential, cocaine may pose a substantially greater danger to ACOAs than alcohol or other drugs. For example, an ACOA who has been able to drink alcohol moderately without problems may conclude, incorrectly, that he/she did not inherit the vulnerability for chemical addiction. With this sense of false confidence, he/she may be receptive to offers of cocaine only to find that the drug compul-sion develops very rapidly. With an estimated 28 million children of alcohol-ics in the U.S. today, the potential for widespread addiction resulting from contact with cocaine is quite real.

CULTURAL FORCES

Cocaine fits in very well with the tenor of our times. For decades now our society has cultivated themes of self-actualization, hedonism, immediate gratification, and narcissistic self-indulgence. "Pleasure now, pay later" ap-pears to be a guiding principle for many. Advertising campaigns promote a "quick fix" mentality. Television dramas and soap operas show grave person-al problems being solved completely within the span of 30 minutes or less. Over-the-counter medicines offer quick relief for minor ailments and annoy-ances, promoting the belief that there should be "a pill to cure every ill." We are all led to believe that we simply should not have to endure or suffer even the most minor discomfort. We expect technology to provide us with the instant solution. "Better living through chemistry" has finally become a reality—we now have an unprecedented menu of potent mood-altering sub-stances, both legal and illegal, for manipulating our brain chemistry into a vast array of desired states.

Perhaps society is changing so fast that people just can't keep up with it all. Disabling stress, depersonalization in an increasing impersonal society, the lack of acceptable goals and values, the breakdown of the family system as the buffer between society and the individual—all of these factors, and more, make cocaine the perfect drug for our times.

COCAINE AND SEX

The so-called "sexual revolution," with its resulting emphasis on sexual freedom, sexual expressiveness, and sexual adventurousness, has also helped to make cocaine a timely plaything. Cocaine has long been touted as an aphrodisiac for enhancing sexual pleasure. For some, the possibility of "missing out" on this type of fun creates a temptation that is just too much to resist. Many but not all users find that cocaine stimulates sexual desire and sexual fantasies and enhances sexual performance, perhaps through a combination of increased desire, decreased inhibitions, and greater physical endurance. Sometimes these effects facilitate or enable sexual experimentation, including group sex, mate swapping, bisexual encounters, and homosexual encounters, in users who report either a lack of desire for these activities or an inability to act on their desire (inhibition) in the absence of cocaine.

Marathon binges of cocaine and sex with multiple partners are not uncommon among those who are dependent on the drug—especially among male freebase smokers. Cocaine can precipitate or fuel a preexisting sexual compulsion, which may manifest itself as compulsive masturbation, multiple encounters, voyeurism, exhibitionism, and other compulsive sexual behaviors.

AVAILABILITY AND AFFLUENCE

Cocaine is available today in sufficient quantities to satisfy the existing demand and at a cost that is no longer prohibitive to an increasing segment of the population. Only a few years ago, when the drug was prohibitively expensive, its use was restricted to the wealthy and elite. Cocaine was a disease of the rich. Few others could afford to indulge or get addicted. Now that virtually anyone can afford it (especially with the appearance of crack), virtually everyone has the opportunity to get addicted to it, and its use is found at all levels of society. Cocaine has truly become an "equal opportunity drug" and cocaine addiction has become an "equal opportunity disease." Nonetheless, affluence can still be a liability when it comes to cocaine. Like monkeys, some people will consume as much as they can get. The more they have, the more they use. Only exhaustion, debilitation, confinement, bankruptcy, or death can eventually stop them.

PREVAILING MYTHS

Despite recent publicity emphasizing the dangers and horrors of cocaine, most users prefer to trust their own experience with the drug. For those in the early "honeymoon" stage of use, anti-drug ads are often perceived as foolish and exaggerated — scare tactics like the "reefer madness" films from days of old. For many who experience the pleasures of cocaine, nothing untoward has happened to them — yet. Therefore they are likely to promote and advertise the fun and safety of cocaine among friends and acquaintances. Positive reports spread quickly in the drug subculture, especially among youth. These reports support the prevailing belief that cocaine is relatively benign and nonaddictive, especially for those who "just" snort it and avoid smoking or injecting it. Now newspaper headlines emphasize crack as the new menace, diverting most of the negative attention away from the dangers of snorting cocaine powder — still the "gateway" form of cocaine for the vast majority of new users.

ADVERSE EFFECTS OF COCAINE

Medical Complications

The potential medical complications of cocaine use are numerous. Cocaine affects many different organ systems and thus the potential for serious physical harm arising from acute or chronic cocaine use can take many different forms. Luckily, for most cocaine users, such complications are still pretty rare. Nonetheless, serious and even tragic consequences of cocaine use do indeed occur, including unpredictable fatal reactions in young and well-conditioned athletes (as evidenced by the deaths of Len Bias and Don Rogers). But most cocaine addicts who seek treatment show little or no evidence of serious or irreversible physical harm, at least insofar as standard medical methods of evaluation are able to detect. As discussed in more detail below, the real danger of cocaine lies not so much in its potential to cause physical harm, but in its unique ability to take control of the user's brain function in a way that malignantly distorts his/her behavior and personality.

Since this book focuses primarily on treating cocaine addiction rather than cocaine-induced medical complications; the latter will be discussed only briefly. Table 2.1 lists some of the most serious medical problems associated with cocaine use. These problems fall into three main categories: (1) overdose or toxic reactions; (2) complications associated with a particular route of cocaine administration; and (3) complications associated with cocaine use during pregnancy.

Exactly how much cocaine must be used and over what period of time in order to cause any of these problems simply cannot be predicted accurately for a particular user. In general, however, higher doses and longer periods of use increase the likelihood of cocaine-related medical problems. An exception is the uncommon but known occurrence of severe or fatal reactions in onetime or occasional users.

DEATH FROM COCAINE

The number of deaths attributed to cocaine use remains relatively small, given the total number of people who use the drug. For example, in 1985 there were 629 reported deaths from cocaine in the U.S. It is likely, however, that this number is an underestimation of the problem. When someone dies of a heart attack or other serious medical problem, the victim's blood or urine is rarely tested for cocaine. Hospital staff may not even be aware that a patient admitted for a serious or even fatal medical condition has been using cocaine—especially if no one mentions it.

Still, even considering the possibility of underreporting, the number of people who actually die from cocaine use remains small. However rare,

TABLE 2.1
Medical Complications From Cocaine

I. **Overdose or Toxic Reactions**
   a. Rapid and/or irregular heartbeat (tachycardia, arrhythmia)
   b. Cardiac arrest (heart attack, ventricular fibrillation)
   c. Cerebral hemorrhage (stroke)
   d. Brain seizure (convulsion with loss of consciousness)
   e. Respiratory failure (suffocation)
   f. Hyperthermia (heat stroke due to elevated body temperature)

II. **Complications Associated with Route of Administration**
   Intranasal
   a. Nasal sores, bleeding, congestion, and discharge
   b. Sinus congestion and headaches
   c. Perforation of the nasal septum

   Freebase Smoking
   a. Chest congestion, wheezing, and black phlegm
   b. Chronic coughing
   c. Lung damage
   d. Burns of the lips, mouth, tongue, and throat
   e. Hoarseness

   Intravenous
   a. Infections at injection sites
   b. Systemic infections (hepatitis, endocarditis, septicemia)
   c. AIDS

III. **Complications From Cocaine Use During Pregnancy**
   a. Premature separation of the placenta; spontaneous abortion
   b. Neurobehavioral deficits in the fetus
   c. Malformation of the fetus
   d. Premature birth, stillbirth, and/or low birth weight

though, the possibility of death from cocaine is nonetheless frightening because it is utterly unpredictable. There is no reliable "safe dose" for any single user. Death has occurred in chronic heavy users as well as first-time users, in low-dose users as well as high-dose users, in snorters and freebase smokers as well as IV users.

The term "overdose," in fact, is misleading because it implies that below some prespecified dose, the use of the drug is relatively safe and toxic or "overdose" reactions can be avoided. Whenever someone has a serious toxic reaction to a drug, it is, by definition, an "overdose," even if the dosage taken is considered by accepted standards to have been fairly small. The same person may react differently to the same dose of cocaine taken on different occasions.

A very small number of people are unable to tolerate any dose of cocaine, owing to a congenital deficiency of the enzyme, pseudocholinesterase, which metabolizes or inactivates cocaine in the blood. Unfortunately, however, people with this congenital deficiency are hardly ever aware of it. For them, one "experiment" with cocaine can be deadly.

There are several ways a user may increase his or her risk of overdosing. One is binge use, taking in an extremely high amount of cocaine over a relatively short period of time. Another is by smoking freebase or crack. Smoking cocaine delivers an extremely high concentration of the drug into the brain very quickly. A third is the use of unusually pure or "uncut" cocaine in a way that far exceeds the user's preexisting tolerance level. While high purity cocaine is more of a rarity than many users realize, cocaine dealers and their close associates often do have access to uncut or lightly cut cocaine. Finally, certain drug combinations tend to increase the chance of causing respiratory or cardiac failure, among them the "speedball" combination of cocaine and heroin.

Cocaine users with certain types of preexisting medical conditions, whether diagnosed or "silent," may be particularly susceptible to fatal reactions. These include people with a history of heart attacks, angina, high blood pressure, and seizure disorders, as well as those who may have underlying but as yet undiagnosed vulnerabilities (partially clogged arteries, minor heartbeat abnormalities, weak spots in artery walls, etc.) which, under the added stress imposed by cocaine, give rise to medical catastrophe.

Signs that a toxic dose may have been ingested include sweating or chills, nausea and vomiting, elevated blood pressure, dilated pupils, tachycardia, delirium, hyperactivity, manic behavior, convulsions, loss of consciousness, and rapid shallow breathing. All such overdose reactions require emergency medical intervention and sometimes life support maneuvers.

Death from cocaine use can also result from contracting the virus that causes acquired immune deficiency syndrome, or AIDS, a risk intravenous users run when they share hypodermic needles. Since 50 to 60 percent of the IV drug users in New York City alone are believed to be already infected with the virus, it is clear that sharing needles can end up being suicidal.

HOW COCAINE KILLS

Fatal reactions to cocaine can occur by a variety of mechanisms. Cocaine can have profound effects on cardiovascular functioning. Its effects on the sympathetic nervous system can cause an increase in heartbeat and blood pressure as well as a constriction or narrowing of blood vessels in the heart and brain. Its local anesthetic effects can change conduction pathways through the heart muscle. These effects, either alone or in combination with one another, can cause sudden death by cardiac arrest and/or stroke. Cocaine can also precipitate grand mal seizures (epileptic convulsions), and sometimes several seizures in rapid succession, which can result in respiratory arrest and death by suffocation. Chronic users may become more sensitive rather than more tolerant to cocaine's seizure-inducing effects (a phenomenon known as "kindling"). As a result of "kindling," use of the same dose may cause no toxic reaction on one occasion and then a totally unexpected and sudden fatal reaction on the next. Cocaine can severely upset the brain regulatory mechanisms that control body temperature. This may lead to hyperthermia (extraordinarily high fevers) and ultimately to convulsions and death.

COCAINE USE DURING PREGNANCY

No level of cocaine use is safe for a pregnant woman or her fetus. Cocaine constricts blood vessels in the umbilical cord and placenta, reducing the supply of oxygen and vital nutrients to the unborn child. The blood supply to the placenta itself may be reduced to the point where it separates from the wall of the uterus (abruptio placentae), sometimes causing a spontaneous abortion or miscarriage. Because the drug crosses the placental barrier as well as fetal blood-brain barrier, the fetus becomes a passive, involuntary recipient of cocaine—sometimes receiving large doses of the drug over long periods of time.

It is of little surprise, therefore, that so-called "cocaine babies," born to mothers who have used cocaine during pregnancy, show an increased incidence of at least several medical complications, including: low birth weight, neurobehavioral deficits, extreme irritability, tremulousness, and insomnia.

While the long-term effects of intrauterine cocaine exposure are still largely unknown, studies suggest that toddlers who were exposed to cocaine in utero exhibit developmental lags, neurological deficits, and behavior problems. Researchers predict that many of these children will be learning disabled and suffer impaired motor skills.

Behavioral and Psychosocial Consequences

The real danger of cocaine use for most people is not death or irreversible physical damage but addiction and dysfunction. The trap for cocaine users lies in the drug's extraordinarily high addictive potential — its ability to chemically control, disrupt, and distort the user's behavior, mood, mental state, and value system, often to the point of dysfunction and serious harm to job, career, and family. The "fallout" from cocaine addiction and its effect on others often provide the major impetus for the addict to seek help. These effects are also responsible for the tremendous toll that cocaine use is having on society at large.

With increasing cocaine involvement, the chronic user may become increasingly irritable, depressed, short-tempered, distractible, unmotivated, reclusive, unreliable, manipulative, demanding, hostile, argumentative, unsociable, erratic, lethargic, paranoid, asexual, suicidal, and ultimately incapable of functioning on a day-to-day basis. Cocaine can cause extreme irritability, paranoia, aggressiveness, and volatility, markedly heightening the user's proclivity toward physical violence. Unfortunately, early warning signs of an individual's involvement with cocaine are often unreliably present and easily overlooked. Clear-cut evidence of regular cocaine use is often not seen until the problem has progressed to the point of serious abuse or addiction.

Because cocaine's cravings are so powerful as to override even basic survival instincts, it is no surprise that the user's basic values and responsibilities are often displaced by this powerful addiction. When the cocaine addict is in the midst of his/her destructive love affair with cocaine, nothing else matters as much as the drug — not family, not friends, not job, sometimes not even life itself. Once the compulsive search for cocaine has been triggered by repeated biochemical alterations in brain activity, obtaining and using cocaine tend to take priority over everything else in the user's life. But these changes in values and behavior are not due, as often assumed, to an inherent unworthiness or sociopathy in the person who becomes addicted. The person may be caring, considerate, and altruistic before the onset of cocaine addiction, but eventually the drug-induced biochemical changes in brain function cause drastic changes in personality and behavior.

The cocaine user's family, friends, and other close relationships can be ravaged by the problem. The chronic user grows increasingly withdrawn from relationships with those who don't use drugs, preferring to be with users or alone, particularly if his or her drug involvement is still a secret from spouse or other family members.

Because of the very high cost of maintaining a cocaine addiction, some users become small-time dealers to offset the cost of their own use. They may sell to friends and acquaintances in order to generate enough profits to pay for their own use. Some become enamored with the easy money from cocaine dealing and make it their main livelihood, giving up good jobs with paychecks that simply can't compete with the money generated from dealing.

Employers and coworkers are also among those affected by the cocaine user's behavioral changes. The user often has a pattern of chronic lateness and absenteeism (especially after holidays and weekends), deteriorating performance levels, and troubled relationships with supervisors and coworkers. Of particular concern are cocaine users who hold jobs that affect public safety. Being actively intoxicated, in the crash state, preoccupied with drug cravings, or physically depleted from a marathon cocaine binge can easily jeopardize innocent nonusers as well as the addicts themselves. Some cocaine users are employed in critical job positions where they are responsible for the health and safety of others: airline pilots, air traffic controllers, train conductors and signal operators, surgeons, nurses, school bus drivers, and nuclear power plant workers — just to name a few. The potential for disaster is obvious.

The risk of serious automobile accidents may be increased by cocaine, especially when it is combined with alcohol or other depressant drugs. Someone who is high on cocaine can usually consume a large amount of alcohol without feeling any of the usual intoxicating, depressant effects. This is because cocaine, a potent but short-acting stimulant, temporarily counteracts alcohol's depressant effects. Since he doesn't feel drunk, the intoxicated cocaine user may be perfectly willing to drive a car. Only a short while later, however, the brief effects of cocaine wear off rapidly and without warning, causing the driver to become almost instantaneously impaired or to fall unconscious. Without opposition from cocaine, the delayed high-dose alcohol effects take over.

In light of the various and substantial risks involved in cocaine use, it becomes apparent that much more is involved in a patient's continuing use of the drug than just the lure of the high or failure to understand the potential risks and consequences. Indeed, for those whose drug compulsion is triggered by repeated cocaine use and its resulting impact on brain chemistry, the drive to get and use more of the drug becomes something outside of the volitional, decision-making process. Like a vehicle on "automatic pilot," the drug-taking behavior becomes self-propelling and self-perpetuating.

Psychiatric Consequences

A common side effect of chronic cocaine use is severe depression. Cocaine-induced depression is evidenced by the same classic symptoms seen in non-drug-related depressions, including: negative moods, lethargy, sleep and appetite problems, anhedonia (inability to experience any pleasure), blunted affect, and suicidal ideation. The "roller-coaster" effect of cocaine's "high-crash" cycle can easily mimic the manic and depressive phases characteristic of bipolar disorders.

Panic attacks, characterized by intense feelings of impending doom, loss of control, confusion, fear, and anxiety, are another common psychiatric consequence of using cocaine. Unpredictable in their onset, these attacks can occur at almost any time, while the user is actively high on cocaine, crashing from cocaine, or abstinent from cocaine between episodes of use.

Lastly, the most serious and clearly the most dangerous psychiatric complication of cocaine use is cocaine psychosis—a serious mental condition characterized by extreme paranoia, suspiciousness, agitation, irritability, social withdrawal, and potentially suicidal or violent behavior. This condition is virtually indistinguishable from a classic paranoid psychosis, including delusions and hallucinations. A person suffering from cocaine psychosis will often feel convinced, despite indisputable objective evidence to the contrary, that close friends and family members are untrustworthy, insincere, and secretly plotting his/her demise. He/she may be reclusive, suicidal, and easily provoked to violence.

Fortunately, in the vast majority of cases, all of the aforementioned cocaine-induced psychiatric complications are temporary and tend to dissipate within a few days after cessation of the drug use. Cocaine-induced depression, however, can persist for as long as several weeks. Most of the psychiatric consequences of cocaine use are not very responsive to standard psychotropic medications used to treat the non-drug-related variety of these disorders. Antidepressants do not appear to relieve cocaine-induced depression. Similarly, antipsychotic medications do not reliably eliminate cocaine-induced psychosis. In most cases, the best treatment is total abstinence from cocaine and all other mood-altering drugs. There are few, if any, reliable ways to predict which cocaine users are most likely to experience serious psychiatric complications. Like other adverse reactions, the onset of drug-induced psychiatric problems is partly a function of the dose and chronicity of use, but even low-dose short-term users can experience these effects. The occurrence of serious psychiatric complications caused by cocaine is a dramatic demonstration of how severely the drug disrupts brain function.

CHAPTER 3

The Addicted Brain

Is COCAINE PHYSICALLY addictive? Does it really cause physical, not just psychological, dependency?

The answer is an emphatic *yes*, even though the cocaine addict does not experience a dramatic withdrawal syndrome. Unlike heroin, the physical addiction to cocaine appears not in the form of withdrawal sickness demanding instant relief from physical pain, but as intense urges and cravings for cocaine that drive the addict to seek out and use the drug time and time again. To say that this acquired drug hunger is due to a process of psychological rather than physical dependency is to ignore some basic biological facts about how mood-altering drugs affect the human brain. Foremost is the fact that in order to produce euphoria or other desired changes in the user's mood and mental state, the drug must get into the user's brain and then penetrate certain brain cells to acutely alter the chemical activity within them. Only those drugs that are capable of altering the biochemical activity of certain brain cells are capable of producing these changes in a person's mood and feeling state.

Of course, it stands to reason that chronic use of any mood-altering drug will ultimately cause chronic changes in the biochemical functioning of affected brain cells. These chronic changes may give rise to compulsive cravings for the drug, impaired cognitive abilities, and negative mood states, all of which will tend to fuel repeated drug use. In a very real sense, then,

35

chronic drug use is a neurological insult to the user's brain with damaging effects that persist beyond the period of intoxication.

It remains to be seen whether the damage is reversible, partially reversible, or permanent. We do know that strong cocaine cravings and mood disorders can sometimes persist in a recovering cocaine addict for many months after stopping all drug use. It seems likely that, at the very least, several months of complete and total abstinence from all psychoactive addictive drugs is required to allow the brain to heal itself from the neurological insult and disruption caused by chronic cocaine use. It seems unlikely that the damage done by chronic cocaine use to the intricate and complicated workings of the human brain can be instantly reversed simply by swallowing a pill.

As might be expected, pharmacologic "cures" and "magic bullets" for cocaine addiction are already being touted by clinicians and enterprising entrepreneurs, now that some of the underlying physiological mechanisms involved in cocaine addiction are being discovered. Although there is nothing wrong with the appropriate time-limited medical use of nonpsychoactive, nonaddictive medications that might relieve some of the post-cocaine symptoms and thereby make it easier for a recovering cocaine addict to achieve or maintain early abstinence, it is important not to create unrealistic expectations which only foster the addict's unhealthy reliance on chemical coping strategies and chemical cures. No medication can substitute for a solid treatment and recovery program which focuses on behavioral, attitudinal, and lifestyle change as the core of recovery from cocaine addiction.

Since cocaine cravings are not accompanied by acute physical discomfort, in the past they were seen merely as evidence of a purely psychological addiction. So it was believed that anyone who really wanted to stop using cocaine could do so quite easily, simply by exerting personal restraint and willpower. Now it is clear that the intense cravings for cocaine have a physiological basis and are not under purely volitional control. Animal studies show that cocaine use can indeed cause a physical addiction equal in power and tenacity to heroin, the drug that most Americans deem the quintessential addictive substance.

THE PROCESS OF ADDICTION

If a drug produces a clear-cut withdrawal syndrome when regular use is discontinued, the presence of painful or annoying withdrawal symptoms may be one factor that contributes to continued use, but these symptoms are neither a necessary nor a sufficient condition to produce or maintain compulsive drug use. Heroin addicts do not take heroin simply to stave off withdrawal. With the benefit of recent knowledge, the long-standing distinction between physical and psychological addiction now seems artificial and invalid. No drug can become psychologically compelling without there being physical (indeed cellular) changes in brain activity that both result from and contribute to its repeated use. Therefore, all mood-altering drugs are physically addicting, even if abrupt discontinuation of use causes no physical withdrawal symptoms.

The Reward Center

A part of the brain thought to be most affected by cocaine is the brain's "reward" center, an area located in the hypothalamus which mediates our basic survival-oriented drives — the ones for food, water, and sex. Repeated introduction of cocaine into this area appears to cause specific changes in neurotransmitter activity, resulting in what amounts to biochemical "misprogramming" of behavior. The drive to use cocaine becomes reinforced in the reward center in much the same way that our other basic drives are.

That may be one reason why, to the cocaine-addicted person, obtaining and using the drug becomes more important than virtually all other involvements, possessions, or activities, including family, health, and career. Any clinician who has treated cocaine addicts has had ample opportunity to observe the devastation: marriages break up, jobs are lost, and finances are depleted in the course of the addict's obsessive and destructive "love affair" with cocaine. An estimated two million Americans, in fact, are already addicted, and an additional six million today are using cocaine regularly (at least once a month), placing themselves in the pool of users most at risk of becoming addicted. Clearly, the most predictive behavioral risk factor for cocaine dependence is repeated use. Perhaps anyone who uses the drug over a long enough period of time and in sufficient doses will trigger off the addictive process in their brain — some at lower doses or with less frequent use than others.

So why do so many people continue to gamble with their own health and life by using cocaine occasionally? Because cocaine is an extraordinarily potent and seductive reinforcer. Laboratory experiments in animals have demonstrated just how easily cocaine can override even the most basic, instinctual biological drives, including the basic instinct to survive. Consider the following observations:

- Hungry monkeys given the choice of cocaine or food almost invariably choose cocaine, ultimately dying of starvation or drug overdose.
- Sex-deprived male monkeys given the choice of pressing a bar for cocaine injections or having sex with a receptive female monkey invariably choose cocaine.

- Rats given unlimited access to cocaine self-administer such massive quantities of the drug that 90 percent die from drug overdose within 30 days. By comparison, with unlimited access to heroin, only 36 percent of rats kill themselves from an overdose within 30 days.
- Monkeys given the choice of pressing a bar to receive a high dose of cocaine followed immediately by an extremely painful electrical shock or of pressing a different bar to receive a much smaller dose of cocaine with no shock invariably opt for the high dose. As the intensity of the shock is increased, the monkeys will continue to choose the high dose, to the point of convulsions and death.

In humans it appears that some people may have a greater biological susceptibility to addiction than others, an issue discussed at length in Chapter 4. But no one is completely immune to addiction, particularly with a drug having such powerfully reinforcing effects as cocaine.

Conditioned Cravings

An important factor contributing to both the development and the maintenance of compulsive cocaine use is conditioned or "learned" cravings for cocaine. When cocaine is used regularly, any person, place, thing, or experience reliably paired or associated with the drug acquires the power to trigger intense cocaine cravings. Almost anything can become a conditioned cue or trigger for cocaine including: drug paraphernalia (e.g., needles, razor blades, freebase pipes, butane torches, plastic straws, mirrors used to lay out "lines," stash boxes used to hide drug supplies); the image of cocaine in a magazine or on a TV screen; the room or building in which cocaine was purchased or used; other people with whom the user has gotten high; a song associated with cocaine use; and even the mere mention of the word "cocaine." Any of these conditioned cues can set off immediate, powerful cravings for cocaine which in turn lead to actual drug use, as illustrated in the following example.

Jerry, a 29-year-old cocaine freebase addict, had achieved eight weeks of total abstinence from all mood-altering substances with the help of our outpatient treatment program and attendance at Cocaine Anonymous meetings. He experienced no spontaneous cravings for cocaine after his first week of abstinence and had discarded all drug paraphernalia from his home and office in an attempt to minimize his exposure to cues that might set off his desire for cocaine. He also avoided bars and nightclubs where he had gotten high on alcohol and cocaine. Since he had not been plagued with obsessive thoughts about cocaine, Jerry was caught "off guard" when his former cocaine dealer called one evening to ask Jerry why he hadn't heard from him in a long while.

From the very instant that Jerry heard the dealer's voice, he became over-whelmed with intense cravings and urges for cocaine and could think of noth-ing else. His heart began to beat rapidly, he felt extremely confused and nervous — even a little nauseous. He became obsessed with thoughts of co-caine. He went immediately to the dealer's home, determined to stay there for only an hour or two. He stayed for three days on a marathon cocaine smoking binge.

Considering the power and pervasiveness of cocaine triggers in the ad-dict's environment, these conditioned responses become an important part of an individual's addiction problem. Achieving and maintaining abstinence from cocaine, therefore, become all but impossible unless the person learns to utilize specific strategies to avoid and cope with cocaine triggers and reminders.

Intense cravings may be more of a factor in cocaine addiction than in other drug addictions, precisely because cocaine's action in the brain occurs in the very same area where basic drives are reinforced. If cocaine were indeed a substance needed for survival, cravings for it would have an adap-tive function, as would being attuned through associative conditioning to all the things that signal "cocaine."

BASIC BRAIN CHEMISTRY

To better understand this process of addiction, let's explore the basics of brain functioning and then how this functioning is affected by drugs such as cocaine. (However, please keep in mind that, particularly with regard to the effects of cocaine on brain mechanisms, the material presented here is a synthesis of current research which at present must be considered merely a "best guess" about how cocaine works in the brain.)

Within the brain networks of neurons (nerve cells) relay all incoming and outgoing information. Different neurons perform different functions. Sen-sory neurons receive information from both internal sources (hormonal levels, temperature, and the like) and external sources (sights, sound, smell, and so on). Interneurons, those with which we are most concerned here, process data received from the sensory neurons and transmit appropriate responses to motor neurons, which control muscle movement and glandular activity. In other words, interneurons receive information from both the body and the environment, interpret it, and dictate a behavioral response.

Let's look at an example. If a man heard and saw a boulder rolling down a hill toward him, his sensory neurons would instantly relay this information to the brain, where it would be processed by interneurons as "danger"; instructions to run like heck would be instantly wired via motor neurons to his legs. An example of a more routine transmission of information would be a person feeling hungry and then walking to the refrigerator to get something to eat. In this case, the sensory neuron receives its cue from internal information (hunger). Data are conveyed to the brain's interneurons for processing and messages dictating behavior conveyed back to the motor neurons.

Each neuron in the brain is positioned among many others so that it can receive and send information from and to various parts of the body. Neurons have many dendrites, or branches, at one end; these receive the incoming information and transfer it to the body of the cell, the axon, where it is processed and transmitted down the length of the cell. Outgoing messages are then sent out via synaptic knobs, or boutons, enlargements at the ends of the axon.

There is a microscopic space between each neuron known as the synapse. It is here that interneural transmission actually takes place (and here that cocaine has its greatest effect). Messages are conveyed across the synapse from one neuron to the next via naturally secreted chemical compounds called neurotransmitters. These electrically charged substances cross the synapse and attach to receptors specific to them on the dendrite of receiving (postsynaptic) neuron. They transmit their message by altering the electrical balance of the receiving neuron, prompting a potential difference, or electrical impulse, to fire the message down the axon of the cell. This process is called an action potential, or simply a nerve impulse. Billions of these exchanges of information are occurring at any given time in the brain.

About 30 different brain neurotransmitters have been identified, but biologists believe there are more yet to be discovered. They are stored in tiny sacs or vesicles in the synaptic knobs, where they can be released into the synapse. Each neurotransmitter appears to specialize in transmitting a particular type of information along specific networks of neurons. The neurotransmitter acetylcholine, for example, transmits messages between motor neurons and skeletal muscles. Norepinephrine plays a key role in orchestrating the body's "fight or flight" response to danger or stress. Serotonin is the neurotransmitter thought chiefly to mediate states of sleep and wakefulness. Endorphins, a recently discovered subgroup of neurotransmitters, are associated with mediating pain and mood by suppressing the flow of certain messages along particular brain circuits. (Morphine and other opiate-derived drugs have been found to resemble endorphins, which may explain why these drugs have found ready receptors in the brain and why the brain is so sensitive to their action.)

Once a neurotransmitter has done its job of carrying the nerve impulse across the synapse to the receptor of the postsynaptic neuron, it is ordinarily released back into the synaptic gap and either metabolized by specific enzymes or reabsorbed by the presynaptic neuron in what is called a reuptake process. In either case the electrical action of the neurotransmitter is extinguished so that the message doesn't keep firing.

All drugs that alter our mood, mental state, or perceptions do so because they are in some way affecting and altering this intricate exchange of chemical impulses. We are only beginning to understand exactly how various drugs affect the process. We know, for instance, that opiate drugs bind themselves to postsynaptic receptors and block the normal transmission of messages regarding pain. Some drugs, such as LSD, psilocybin, and mescaline, cause hallucinations—obviously by affecting brain neural transmissions, but in ways not yet understood. Preliminary studies suggest that alcohol may inhibit the neurotransmitter serotonin and enhance the action of another, γ-aminobutyric acid, thought to help relieve anxiety. (Alcohol also kills about 10,000 neurons with every ounce consumed, probably accounting for the loss of mental acuity seen in some chronic alcoholics.)

Cocaine's Effect on Dopamine

Dopamine is thought to be the most important neurotransmitter involved in stimulating nerve-impulse transmissions within the brain's reward center. Under normal conditions, a certain amount of dopamine is naturally released from the presynaptic vesicles as needed to maintain a normal mood and mental state and to reinforce the satisfaction of normal drives with a sense of pleasure we call satiation. Once the dopamine reaches a receptor on the postsynaptic neuron, the enzyme acetylcholinesterase acts to neutralize it, extinguishing its chemically coded message. The receptor, in effect, "gets the message," and then the dopamine is broken down so that the message is not sent repeatedly. Finally, extra dopamine that has not connected with a receptor but remains in the synapse is carried back by another enzyme into the neuron that released it, through the reuptake process already described. There it is stored until it is needed for another release.

Cocaine use significantly alters virtually every aspect of the normal neural transmission process. Keep in mind, however, that very little is known for certain about how cocaine affects neurotransmitter activity and that what is presented here must be considered a best guess based on current knowledge, most of which has been extrapolated from animal studies. What we don't know yet about how cocaine (and other drugs) affect the brain amounts to much more than what we do know—and therein lies one good reason for avoiding their use altogether. Based on what little is known, however, it appears that cocaine alters neurotransmissions in the following manner.

First, when cocaine is present, the neurons are stimulated to release a flood of dopamine, much more than they would ordinarily. To supply this stepped-up release, the brain also begins to produce greater initial stores of dopamine. Since dopamine is thought to transmit feelings of pleasure and well-being, this greater output of dopamine could account for the touted euphoria provided by cocaine. This accelerated release is also one factor that causes the neuron to eventually become depleted of dopamine.

Second, to accommodate the increased flow of dopamine into the neural synapse, neurons develop additional dendrites or branches on the post-synaptic end, thus providing more receptors to receive the extra dopamine. (These extra receptors probably contribute to the development of tolerance.) There are now more dopamine-specific receptors to be satisfied than before, requiring that more dopamine be released, which in turn requires more cocaine. The overall effect is to contribute to the developing drug hunger, concomitant with a decreasing ability to satisfy receptors sufficiently to provide the high — driving the user further and further into compulsive use. Third, cocaine causes the neural impulse to keep firing in the synapse, probably contributing to the exhilaration, euphoria, and stimulant effects of cocaine. This is also why, in high doses, cocaine (and amphetamines too) can cause such an overload of firing that the messages transmitted from the brain to other parts of the body become chaotic. Convulsions possibly resulting in death may occur when brain mechanisms controlling heart function or respiration are affected.

The reason why the impulse keeps firing when cocaine induces a release of dopamine is that the drug destroys the enzyme that ordinarily extinguishes the chemical message carried by the dopamine. As a result, the neuron continues to be stimulated by this molecule of dopamine that has attached itself to the receptor and continues firing for a period of time in the synapse.

Finally, cocaine also destroys the enzyme that carries any remaining dopamine back into the nerve cell that released it. In other words, it blocks the reuptake process. The extra dopamine remains, then, in the synaptic gap, leaving the presynaptic neuron temporarily short of its supply.

THE COCAINE CRASH

The cocaine crash is thought to be due to this temporary dopamine shortage. It takes time for the neurons to manufacture more of these neurotransmitters. Since dopamine is essential to maintaining a normal mood and mental state, this temporary shortage results in a crash, typically lasting from 30 to 60 minutes or more.

During this time the user typically feels tired, anxious, depressed, irritable, and unable to sleep. What the brain really needs is to rest and synthesize more dopamine, but it has been chemically misprogrammed into craving more cocaine instead. The crash reinforces the cycle of continued use since ingesting more cocaine provides immediate relief from its symptoms.

The aftereffects of most drugs are dose-dependent, and cocaine's crash (again, like alcohol's hangover) is no exception. While the amount of cocaine it takes to cause a crash varies from person to person, generally speaking, the higher the high from cocaine, the more intense the crash. People who use small amounts of cocaine at infrequent intervals may not experience any crash at all, so it may not be an important factor in motivating their further use. In freebase smokers and IV users, however, because of the higher dosages of cocaine delivered to the brain, the crash is usually more intense and demands relief obtained either by taking more cocaine or by using other drugs such as alcohol, tranquilizers, sleeping pills, marijuana, or opiates. Accordingly, it is common for cocaine addicts to enter treatment cross-addicted to one or more of these other drugs as well.

TOLERANCE

Tolerance to a drug is evidenced by the need to take increasingly higher doses in order to achieve the same effect. The development of tolerance to cocaine is evidenced by the fact that many chronic users increase their cocaine intake to dosage levels that would have been distinctly toxic or even lethal at earlier stages of use. Chronic high-dose users invariably report no longer experiencing any euphoria at all from their cocaine use, indicating that tolerance to the high develops as well. It is thought that this occurs because the neurons have attempted to accommodate the increased supply of dopamine in the synapse by developing more dendrites (branches) and more receptors.

Even after the high is no longer experienced, addicted users will typically continue compulsively seeking and using the drug, almost as if their drug-using behavior has become reflexive and automatic. This is because cravings for cocaine continue to be generated by the neural circuits of the reward center, which are, in effect, misprogrammed to seek cocaine as a survival need and experiencing a depletion of even their normal amount of dopamine. Added to this is the chronic depression resulting from this depletion, which the user has come to know can be temporarily and partially alleviated by cocaine. Although the drug may no longer result in euphoria, addicted users report that a dose can at least make them feel slightly less depressed and less miserable.

As repeated drug use results in less and less pleasure, the addict becomes most and more compulsive about using the cocaine. Continued use is driven to an increasing extent by the cocaine-induced biochemical alterations in brain function in combination with behavioral and environmental factors that promote habitual drug-taking patterns. At this point the user is in a terrible bind. Taking cocaine is no longer pleasurable, but not taking it feels even worse. Some will become motivated to enter treatment. Others will chase the cocaine high; that is, they will increase their use even further in a desperate attempt to recapture the elusive euphoric effects of cocaine based on vividly recalled memories from an earlier stage of use. Of course, this effort is doomed to failure.

Kindling

With repeated use, tolerance develops to nearly all of cocaine's effects — with one major exception. The ability of cocaine to induce a convulsion or brain seizure may actually increase with continued use. That is, the user may become more, rather than less, sensitive to cocaine's seizure-inducing properties as usage continues. What was once a tolerable dose for a person can become a toxic or even a fatal dose, with no warning whatsoever. Most users don't know about this effect. Because a larger and larger dose of cocaine is required to achieve the same high (due to tolerance), users often assume that they are becoming less sensitive to all of cocaine's effects. This can be a fatal error.

This phenomenon of reverse tolerance is known as the kindling effect. Animal studies suggest that certain neurons in the central nervous system that are repeatedly exposed to cocaine become sensitized to the drug and thus fire more readily with each successive drug exposure. With long-term use these neurons fire even in the presence of relatively low doses of cocaine. The kindling phenomenon may also explain why some chronic users report a selectively increased sensitivity to the unpleasant stimulant effects of cocaine (feelings of nervousness, restlessness, agitation, etc.).

DOPAMINE DEPLETION WITH CHRONIC USE

Because cocaine stimulates cells to discharge much more of their dopamine stores than they would ordinarily, and because the extra dopamine left in the synapse is unable to be reabsorbed, as it would normally be via the reuptake process, the brain cells of chronic cocaine users are eventually depleted of this vital neurotransmitter. Normally, after a non-drug-induced release of dopamine, the cells are able to replenish their supplies by manufacturing more dopamine. But cocaine appears to overtax the system: With frequent cocaine use, cells are simply releasing more dopamine than they are able to replace. This has been compared to a sponge that has been squeezed dry — there is simply no liquid left in it. Cocaine's various effects on neural transmission take place each time the drug is used, but it is this eventual depletion of dopamine that may actually cause the physiological addiction.

Since dopamine appears to be vital to maintaining a normal mood and mental state, a deficiency of it induces dysphoria (the opposite of euphoria) and anhedonia (the inability to experience pleasure normally). Even those activities that would ordinarily bring pleasure—leisure, recreation, sports, sex—can no longer be enjoyed. There is simply too little dopamine remaining in the brain cells to respond to the normal pleasures of life; the reward centers have become refractory to stimulation. Ironically, at this point the user is usually experiencing the opposite of what was initially sought through cocaine use: In place of euphoria there is dysphoria, a chronically negative mood state; instead of an elevated mood one experiences chronic irritability and anxiety; instead of increased energy there is chronic fatigue; in place of greater social ease and spontaneity there are usually bouts of paranoia and an increasing tendency to withdraw socially; perceived increases in mental acuity give way to a shortened attention span, poor concentration, and mental confusion; where there was heightened interest in people and surroundings there is now apathy; any initial increase of sexual interest gives way in many cases to a loss of sexual desire and even impotence.

The user is trapped in a vicious cycle, craving the very drug that is causing the depression. Using cocaine doesn't even bring relief anymore—it only makes matters worse; yet the compulsion to continue using only escalates. Without help, cocaine addicts that reach this state of depression have increased risks of suicide attempts, accidents, and overdoses.

STAGES ON THE ROAD TO ADDICTION

The road to addiction is not clearly marked. The user cannot know when he or she is moving from one stage of use into another, for there is no clearly discernible line separating them. For each person the process will differ a little, depending on the form of cocaine used, potency of the doses, method of administration, and frequency of use. The following outline of stages can serve as a guideline, however, for understanding the progression.

Experimental Use

This type of use tends to be motivated by such factors as curiosity, social encouragement, role-modeling, and the desire to share a presumably pleasant and harmless experience. This is the "honeymoon" stage of cocaine use during which the user experiences only good effects from cocaine. It is at this point that one can easily feel convinced by a purely positive experience with cocaine that all prior warnings about the negative effects and dangers are simply exaggerated and untrue.

Just how long the honeymoon with cocaine lasts is dose-dependent. Those who begin by smoking crack often progress quickly to high doses and skip this first stage altogether, while some infrequent cocaine snorters stay indefinitely in the experimental stage. On the basis of early evidence, however, we can surmise that experimental users who continue to use cocaine run a risk of moving on to the next stage, that of regular use. Not everyone who tries cocaine will do so, of course. Some people consider what they have heard or learned about the drug's harmful effects and opt to stop using it as the best insurance against becoming addicted.

Regular Use

In this stage using cocaine starts to become a regular feature of one's lifestyle. When an experimental user begins routinely to plan to use cocaine whenever an important occasion arises or before every date or at every party, he or she is beginning to move into regular use. It becomes difficult to think of doing certain things or of having a good time without cocaine. The pattern of use may still be intermittent or sporadic, perpetuated by the powerfully rewarding effects of the drug and the absence of any significant negative consequences directly attributable to the drug use. Many still consider this to be recreational use, because even though use is now frequent, users at this stage often still have not begun to suffer any apparent negative consequences, reinforcing the belief that cocaine is harmless — at least for them.

This is actually a very dangerous stage, because the biochemical changes, such as the repeated stimulation of the brain's reward center and resultant dopamine depletion, are beginning to occur. It is possible to be a regular user and not yet be fully addicted, but at some point the invisible line into compulsive use can unwittingly be crossed.

Addictive Use

Once a person no longer has control over cocaine, no longer can choose to use it or not use it, he or she is addicted. The most reliable signs of cocaine addiction are:

(1) Overwhelming urges and cravings for the drug. The addicted user is preoccupied with getting and using cocaine. It has higher priority than any other activity, even though the user may not be getting high anymore.

(2) An inability to self-limit or control use. Someone who is cocaine-dependent can usually stop using cocaine temporarily, for days,

weeks, or months at a time, but finds it impossible to stay away from the drug on a more permanent basis, even with strenuous efforts to exert self-control and willpower. An addict has usually broken many promises to him/herself and others to stop using the drug once and for all.

(3) Continued use of cocaine despite negative consequences to the user's functioning. Cocaine use may continue even in the face of depression, paranoia, suicidal feelings, loss of productivity at work or school, loss of job, financial losses, strained relationships, legal problems, etc.

(4) Denial that the drug use is a problem. The cocaine addict usually downplays the seriousness of the negative effects cocaine is having, denies that there is a problem, and gets angry and defensive if someone suggests that his or her drug use is out of control. At this point the person has probably developed tolerance to cocaine and keeps increasing the dose, both to try to recapture the euphoric high and to stave off both the crash and the intensifying depression resulting from chronic cocaine use.

Because cocaine is commonly used in binges separated by periods of nonuse, it often appears that binge users who are able to abstain for days or weeks at a time are not addicted. It is important to keep in mind that addiction is defined not by the frequency or amount of use, but rather by the role that the drug use plays in the individual's life and by his or her pathological, obsessive relationship with the drug. Some people who snort small amounts of cocaine infrequently seem to demonstrate no signs of addiction or compulsive use. As tolerance develops, however, even the occasional user's brain requires more cocaine for the same high, and somewhere along the line most people increase the amount and frequency of their use—especially if they enjoy the effects. Furthermore, cocaine affects the brain and other organs in increments, so that the addictive process may be set in motion without the user's awareness.

Much remains to be learned about the addicted brain. However, despite the intuitive appeal of physiological explanations for overt behavior, it is not cocaine's biochemical action alone that determines whether an individual becomes addicted to this or any other drug. Several additional factors can be assumed to play an integral part in the etiology of addictive disease, as explored in Chapter 4, "Understanding Addictive Disease."

CHAPTER 4

Understanding Addictive Disease

Is COCAINE ADDICTION really a disease? Academic debates over this question will probably continue for decades. Many people will remain unreceptive to the idea that drug addiction is a disease without scientific evidence of a specific genetic factor predisposing certain people to the problem and discovery of a specific physiological mechanism responsible for its expression. In the absence of such clear-cut evidence, it is likely that addicts (and alcoholics) will, unfortunately, continue to be seen by many as individuals of "weak character" who have voluntarily inflicted the problem on themselves.

Academic debates aside, for purely clinical reasons it can be extremely helpful—to the patient, the family, and the treatment professional—to conceptualize and deal with cocaine addiction as a disease. Although in the final analysis we must all be held responsible for our behavior (no matter what its cause), those who are victims of a disease are generally viewed and treated somewhat differently. People who are deemed to be "sick" rather than "bad" are typically treated with more compassion, tolerance, and concern. Given the popular view of drug addicts as excessive self-indulgers who live in a chemically-induced state of blissful euphoria, it is easy to overlook the pain, suffering, and despair characteristic of the addict's existence. Most addicted individuals have not experienced euphoria or any other pleasurable effects from their drugs for months or years. They no longer get "high" from taking drugs—they become depressed, dysphoric, even suicidal and engage in self-defeating, maladaptive behavior. It is difficult to understand the habitual, self-destructive tendency of the addict who resorts to repeated drug use even in the face of horrendous consequences as anything but pathological.

Most alcoholism treatment is based on the conviction that alcoholism is a disease and the American Medical Association (AMA) has urged physicians to treat it as such since the early 1950s. Among the general public many people still think of the alcoholic as weak or morally deficient, not as someone who is suffering from a chronic and potentially fatal illness that he/she did not elect to have. The continuing controversy on this subject was highlighted in the recent Supreme Court case involving the Veterans Administration's claim that two recovering alcoholic Vietnam veterans were not entitled to extension of their disability benefits because the VA considered their alcoholism to be "willful misconduct" rather than a legitimate medical illness causing temporary disability. Nevertheless, aided in part by scientific studies suggesting that an increased susceptibility to alcoholism can be inherited, more people are coming to accept alcoholism as an illness or condition—something akin to an "allergy" to alcohol.

By contrast, most people (including many treatment professionals) still have difficulty accepting drug addiction as a disease, especially in the case of illegal drug use. But just as we are learning to look beyond the alcoholic's "bad behavior" to the compulsiveness and lack of choice that underlie it, we must begin to apply this new understanding of addiction to cocaine and other illicit drugs as well. Drug abuse treatment professionals as a whole have been slow not only to recognize drug addiction as a disease but also to educate patients about it. Some feel that telling drug addicts that they have a disease will simply give them a convenient excuse for getting high over and over again, a "cop-out" from personal responsibility. This raises a crucial point, namely, that while the addict is not personally responsible for having the disease (i.e., the pathological response to mood-altering drugs), he/she is most certainly responsible for remaining abstinent and working a recovery program. In other words, while the addict cannot control the way he/she reacts to drugs (no more than the hayfever sufferer can control sneezing and watery eyes in response to pollen), the addict can indeed control whether or not he/she makes contact with drugs or puts them into his/her body. With this crucial distinction in mind, accepting one's drug addiction as a permanent, lifelong illness requiring total abstinence in order to arrest the active symptoms, increases rather than decreases personal responsibility.

What does it mean to say that cocaine addiction (or any other chemical addiction for that matter) is a disease? In the literature of Alcoholics Anonymous, chemical dependency is described as a disease consisting of two parts: (1) an allergy of the body and (2) an obsession of the mind. This is another way of saying that the disease has both physical and psychological components. The physical component is thought to include biological factors such as (1) a genetically inherited predisposition to addictive disease and (2) a chemical alteration of brain function caused by the chronic drug use itself that both creates the compulsive desire (cravings) for drugs and disables cognitive abilities and coping skills — the net result being a perpetuation of the drug use. As one might expect, the psychological component of the disease is harder to define. The addict's obsession with drugs is often an outgrowth of attempts to utilize these substances as magical (but totally ineffective) solutions to life's problems. Drugs are used habitually to get rid of negative feelings (e.g., depression, anger, anxiety) that stem from certain problems, but such "chemical coping" does nothing to solve the problems that are eliciting the negative feelings. Inevitably, the problems get worse, the negative feelings intensify, and the drug use escalates in an effort to escape from the ever-worsening predicament. This is the vicious cycle of self-defeating, addictive behavior. It is no wonder, then, that individuals with low frustration tolerance, poor coping skills, and an underdeveloped sense of self, for example, are often highly attracted to drugs that offer the promise of instant correction and relief.

The disease model of addiction has clinical value not only in understanding how the problem might develop, but also in formulating effective treatments. For example, if one accepts that the disease is not the drug use per se but the tendency to resort to compulsive, self-defeating drug use in the face of problems and negative feelings, then abstinence is not the only appropriate goal of treatment. Stopping all drug use is merely the prerequisite for developing alternative coping skills and learning how to recognize and deal with negative feelings more adaptively.

To better understand the disease model, let's utilize the analogy of addictive disease as an allergy. Most people would probably agree on the following points regarding common allergies, such as those to foods, medicines, and other things like grass or trees: (1) The allergic individual is generally not held to be personally at fault or responsible for the fact that the allergy exists and he/she experiences an allergic reaction upon exposure to certain allergens; (2) the allergic individual is expected to have no control over the nature or intensity of his/her physiological reaction to the allergen once the reaction is set off; (3) the allergic individual is expected to exhibit the allergic reaction and its characteristic symptoms every time or almost every time he/she is exposed to the allergen, unless vulnerability can somehow be lowered; and (4) the allergic individual is expected to avoid exposure to the allergen altogether or, at the very least, to minimize exposure to the allergen, if at all possible.

Let us stay with the allergy model for a moment and consider what would happen, for example, if someone severely allergic to feathers denied or minimized the problem and continued to sleep with a down comforter and pillows. He/she would undoubtedly continue to have allergy symptoms. But if this allergic person fully accepted having the allergy (susceptibility) and genuinely desired to be free of allergic symptoms, even at the expense of some personal comfort, then he/she would naturally make behavioral changes and decisions to keep exposure to feathers at an absolute minimum.

Likewise, once a drug addict unquestionably accepts having the chronic (incurable) disease of addiction, then, and only then, will the addicted individual begin consistently to make the kinds of decisions that will support abstinence and recovery. It is paradoxical that only by accepting the lack of control over drug use and its effects on behavior does an individual afflicted with addictive disease begin to acquire some degree of control over his/her life. The starting point is to categorically avoid any exposure whatsoever to the "allergen" which activates the disease, in this case cocaine (and all other mood-altering chemicals).

It is not difficult to see why a thorough and accurate understanding of addictive disease can be extremely helpful to a cocaine-addicted individual who is attempting to recover from the problem. But accepting one's vulnerability, as the disease model requires, is not easy to do in our society, where so much importance is placed on being in control of oneself, being strong, and overcoming problems with sheer determination and willpower. This is the very "pioneer spirit" upon which the country was founded, and these themes remain ever-present in today's culture. No wonder that the inability to admit powerlessness over addiction remains a hurdle in the recovery of so many.

There are at least several distinct benefits to cocaine addicts of accepting their problem as a disease:

(1) It helps to crystallize the rationale for abstaining from all mood-altering drugs. When an addict accepts the existence of his/her vulnerability to drugs and understands that it can be triggered by any drug use whatsoever, he/she will probably be better able to forego any opportunities for use (exposure). The argument of "My problem is with cocaine — not alcohol or marijuana — so I should be able to keep drinking or smoking pot as long as I stay away from cocaine" loses validity when he/she understands that a relapse to cocaine addiction can be triggered by the use of any mood-altering substance whatsoever and that recovery from the addictive disease is impossible as long as drug use of any type continues. It no longer seems as though the treatment program or counselor is simply trying to take away anything

that's fun by applying rigid rules about abstinence arbitrarily and dogmatically. The addict can begin to embrace the need to avoid the broad category of all mood-altering drugs, in much the same way some people must avoid dairy products because their digestive system cannot handle them.

(2) Once the addicted individual accepts that the vulnerability is within him/herself, whether due to inherited predisposition or to repeated drug-taking itself, he/she can begin to accept personal responsibility for making the behavioral and lifestyle changes necessary to achieve and maintain abstinence; by avoiding high-risk situations; by attending to negative mood states that can be precursors to relapse; in short, by doing everything possible to avoid re-exposure to their allergic agent, cocaine, and any other mood-altering drugs.

(3) An understanding that drug addiction is a disease and that loss of control is a symptom of the disease can lift a great burden of guilt from the addict and thereby freeing up more constructive energy to be channeled into recovery rather than self-pity. No longer must he/she harbor unbearable feelings of weakness and worthlessness for having succumbed to addiction. This in turn makes it far easier to admit to and accept the addiction, for now being an addict is not such a self-indictment. One reason for the fierce denial in addiction may be that facing and admitting the problem mean getting in touch with deep-seated feelings of shame related to the stigma of being an addict. Cognitively reframing the addiction problem as a disease that is out of one's own control and for which one is not to blame helps to lessen this stigma. The patient can then more easily say, "I am an addict," without feeling it is synonymous with saying, "I am a bad and worthless person." Commonly heard among recovering people in the rooms of Cocaine Anonymous (CA), Alcoholics Anonymous (AA), and other self-help programs is the saying, "I'm not a bad person getting good but a sick person getting better." For the vast majority of addicts, then, coming to view oneself as a sick person does not become an excuse for staying sick. It becomes a starting place from which to get better.

(4) Recognizing that the disease is both physical and psychological helps the recovering addict see the importance not only of staying off drugs but also of making permanent changes in life-style, attitude, and behavior. Recovery from addictive disease is defined as the process of developing an entirely new, healthier way of living and being.

DISEASE CRITERIA

How can we justify defining chemical dependency, including cocaine addiction, as a disease? Many people balk at the idea of calling addiction a disease, arguing that since addicts have "chosen" to use drugs they should be able to "unchoose" them as well. Also, when the drugs being used are illegal and the user sometimes commits crimes to obtain them, it is difficult for many people to view the addict as sick rather than bad. Compassion and understanding are not easily offered to those who commit antisocial acts.

Insofar as the volitional aspect is concerned, it is hard to imagine that anyone really chooses to have an illness or disease. No one who gets involved with drugs does so with the intention or expectation of becoming an addict. In fact, most beginning users are convinced that they can handle the drugs they choose and that it is simply not within their makeup or personality to become addicted. It must also be recognized that most people who try drugs do not become addicts. Similarly, not all cigarette smokers become cancer victims; not all people exposed to the pathogens for measles, polio, or influenza get those diseases either. For those who do come down with the disease, one can only assume that a pre-existing susceptibility (e.g., perhaps a weakened immune system in the case of infections, or a biochemical reaction in the brain in the case of drug addictions) has played a significant role in determining whether exposure leads to the illness.

Addiction to cocaine (or other drugs) meets accepted criteria for other illnesses more readily acknowledged as diseases. Specifically, cocaine addiction is: (1) diagnosable; (2) primary, and itself the cause of other problems, both medical and psychiatric; (3) predictable and progressive in its course; and (4) treatable.

Diagnosable

Cocaine addiction is not vague or mysterious. It can be recognized and described by certain signs and symptoms and is therefore diagnosable. An experienced health professional can readily and accurately ascertain when the disease is present and when it is not. Further, cocaine addiction can be differentiated from cocaine abuse. The abuser may be experiencing negative effects from using cocaine but has not crossed the line into compulsive use that is outside volitional control. When the cocaine abuser experiences negative consequences from using the drug, he/she either stops or drastically reduces his/her use. When the cocaine addict experiences negative consequences from using the drug, he/she continues or even escalates his/her use. The addict may want to stop using the drug, but finds it impossible to do so without outside help and/or a drastic change in environmental circumstances. As mentioned earlier, the diagnostic signs of addiction include: (1) loss of control over use; (2) cravings and obsession with the drug; (3) continued use despite adverse consequences; and (4) denial that the problem exists even in the face of objective evidence to the contrary.

In terms of describable everyday behavior, the person who is addicted will probably break promises and resolutions to stop or control use; lie about use and otherwise hide it from concerned others; undergo personality changes when high and/or without a drug supply, including mood swings, emotional withdrawal, depression, or suicidal behavior; gravitate toward other compulsive/heavy users as friends and withdraw from non-users; suffer severe problems in intimate relationships, resulting from making cocaine the first priority; have to use larger and larger quantities of the drug just to feel "normal" (that is, develop tolerance); experience less and less pleasure from cocaine yet feel compelled to continue using it anyway; suffer episodes of paranoid psychosis; experience impaired functioning at work or school; and demonstrate increasing chaos in financial affairs, including excessive and uncontrolled spending for cocaine, resulting in the draining of all financial resources, the selling of possessions, and even theft and robbery. Of course, there is a great deal of person-to-person variability in the way that cocaine addiction and its consequences are exhibited. For example, some cocaine addicts show severe deterioration and obvious problems in their psychosocial functioning. Their behavior is erratic, unpredictable, dysfunctional. Other addicts are able to maintain at least a façade of adequate functioning. They strive at all costs to "look good" — to maintain their job, home, and significant relationships — but eventually something gives out and the resulting crisis exposes their dysfunction more clearly.

The psychiatric community has finally given official recognition to the fact that cocaine "dependence" really does exist. The Diagnostic and Statistical Manual (*DSM-III-R*) of the American Psychiatric Association lists specific diagnostic criteria for cocaine dependence. Individuals who exhibit three or more of the following behaviors and diagnostic signs are said to meet the criteria for a diagnosis of cocaine dependence:

1. Cocaine is often taken in larger amounts or over a longer period of time than the user intended.
2. The user has a persistent desire, or has made one or more unsuccessful attempts to cut down or control his/her cocaine use.
3. The user spends a great deal of time in activities necessary to obtain cocaine, use cocaine, or recover from its effects.
4. The user is frequently intoxicated or experiencing post-drug reactions when expected to fulfill major role obligations at work, school, or home, or when cocaine use is physically hazardous (e.g., drives a car while high on cocaine).
5. The user foregoes important social, occupational, or recreational activities because of cocaine use.
6. The user continues to take cocaine despite knowledge that persistent or recurrent social, psychological, or physical problems are being caused or exacerbated by the continued use.
7. The user shows marked tolerance to cocaine evidenced by the need for substantially increased amounts of the drug in order to achieve intoxi-

cation or other desired effects, or shows a markedly diminished effect from continued use of the same amount.

Primary

The disease of cocaine (and other drug) dependency is primary; that is, it is not merely a symptom of another underlying condition or illness and can itself cause secondary medical and psychiatric problems that cannot be effectively treated unless the primary addiction is arrested. Some of the secondary problems associated with cocaine addiction include high blood pressure, insomnia, weight loss, brain seizures, panic attacks, depression, paranoid psychosis, suicidal or homicidal behavior, sexual dysfunction, and psychosocial dysfunction or impairment.

Many clinicians have traditionally viewed drug addiction as secondary to underlying psychological problems. To the extent that certain psychological problems may put a person at increased risk for developing addictive disease, this view is probably accurate. But once the addictive process has occurred in the brain, regardless of what may have contributed to its etiology, the addiction itself becomes primary and must be treated as such.

Progressive and Predictable in Its Course

The disease of cocaine addiction is chronic, never reverses, and grows progressively more severe if left untreated. (The typical progression of addictive disease through early, middle, and late stages is shown in Table 4.1.) By *chronic* we mean that cocaine addiction is never a single acute attack but is marked by permanence, with a continued vulnerability to recurring symptoms (relapse). It can also be terminal.

Perhaps the most baffling observable characteristic of addictive disease is the fact that it continues to exist whether or not the addicted person continues to use the drug. Once a person has the disease, even if he/she is abstinent for a long period of time, the symptoms of addiction will occur again from renewed contact with the drug, often with the same severity as when abstinence was first begun. That is, the relapsed addict generally does not go through a second progressive sequence of gradually increasing use. The renewed usage and its consequences tend to "pick up" at a more advanced stage of the disease progression and escalate rapidly. Addicts get no second "honeymoon" with cocaine. Although the fantasy of returning to the bliss of the early cocaine-induced high often contributes to the allure of resuming cocaine use, that initial euphoria can rarely be recaptured. If the user tries cocaine after a period of abstinence, the cocaine obsession is usually rekindled immediately, compelling the relapsed addict to use again and again. Some relapses are short-lived. Some are extensive. Some are fatal.

TABLE 4.1
The Course of Cocaine Addiction

EARLY STAGE

Brain chemistry altered
Addictive thinking begins
Obsessive thoughts
Compulsive urges
Conditioned cravings
Lifestyle changes
Withdrawal from normal activities
Subtle physical and psychological consequences
  (jitters, irritability, mood swings, etc.)

MIDDLE STAGE

Loss of control
Cravings
Inability to stop despite consequences
Denial
Increasing isolation
Increasing physical and psychological conse-
  quences—paranoia, panic, seizures, etc.
Impaired work/school performance

LATE STAGE

Failure of efforts to stop
Severe financial problems
Severe work/school dysfunction
Plummeting self-esteem
Severe relationship problems
Chronic severe depression
Cocaine psychosis
Death

Treatable

The good news, of course, is that cocaine addiction, like other addictive diseases, is treatable. While it cannot be cured, its symptoms can be arrested by total abstinence from all mood-altering chemicals. Following abstinence, an addict's vulnerability to relapsing can be lowered through permanent changes in life-style, attitude, and behavior. Contrary to the common assumption that addicts are impossible to treat and that successful treatment outcomes are rare, the prognosis in most cases is good to excellent, provided that the addict has a genuine desire to stop using drugs and that certain treatment requirements are met.

WHO IS PRONE TO ADDICTION?

As with any other measure of health, one's vulnerability to chemical addiction lies on a continuum, with none of us entirely invulnerable. A number of factors may contribute to our place on that continuum, some of which can shift during the course of a lifetime, raising or lowering our degree of risk at any given point in time. Addictive disease occurs when a person somehow exceeds his/her invisible and unknown threshold level on the continuum of vulnerability and triggers a certain biochemical response in the brain through repeated drug use.

For the person who starts out high on the vulnerability scale to begin with — owing to the physical, psychological, or environmental factors to be explored in this section — little repeated drug use is needed to set the process in motion. But even the person who starts out low on the scale — who has not inherited genetic predisposition, has not learned drug-coping from family models, and does not suffer from chronic negative mood states — can trigger the addictive response in the brain with repeated use. This is why the widespread acceptance of cocaine use in our society during the 1970s and 1980s resulted in addiction among many people who were previously well-functioning — much to everyone's surprise. A reasonably content, stable person can still become addicted — to alcohol, cocaine, or any other addictive drug — with enough repeated use. Since cocaine's pharmacological qualities make it more likely to cause addiction than many other drugs, a relatively high percentage of those who use cocaine with regularity end up addicted.

Of course, no one can know before experimenting where on the scale of vulnerability he/she is, so no one can (or should) conclude, "I'm not at risk, so I can use cocaine once a month or so without any risk of getting addicted."

There are at least several factors that might contribute to an individual's vulnerability to addictive disease.

Physical Predisposition

One may be more or less vulnerable to addictive disease based on biological inheritance. For example, studies have shown that babies separated from alcoholic parents at birth and raised by non-alcoholic adoptive parents grow up with twice the incidence of alcoholism of babies born to non-alcoholic biological parents and raised by non-alcoholic adoptive parents. These findings suggest that a hereditary factor may contribute to the emergence of alcoholism in at least some cases, and that emergence of the problem cannot be accounted for entirely by the environmental influence of growing up in an alcoholic home. There is, as yet, no evidence of an inherited vulnerability specific to cocaine addiction. In fact, it seems very unlikely that any inherited factor would be drug-specific; that is, there is probably no specific chromosome or gene that is cocaine-specific, alcohol-specific, or heroin-specific, etc. Rather, it seems more likely that what one might inherit is a generalized vulnerability to chemical dependency which could be brought out or triggered by any number of different mood-altering drugs.

At least one study supports this possibility. As mentioned in Chapter 2, a survey of 161 primary cocaine addicts who entered my outpatient treatment program, revealed that nearly half had at least one alcoholic or drug-abusing parent or grandparent. Interestingly, many of these cocaine addicts reported no history of alcohol abuse or alcoholism prior to the onset of their cocaine addiction. This finding suggests that perhaps cocaine—more easily than alcohol—can spark an underlying vulnerability to addiction. Adult children of alcoholics (ACOAs) who find themselves able to drink safely, would be well advised to not conclude from the experience that they have not inherited an increased vulnerability to addiction. Due to its exceptionally high addiction potential, cocaine must be considered an exceptionally dangerous drug to ACOAs.

Psychological Vulnerability

Mainstream psychiatrists, who have long seen drug abuse as a symptom of underlying psychiatric disorder, are certainly not wholly mistaken. There is no doubt that chronic uncomfortable or dysphoric mood states increase one's likelihood to want to try a mood-altering drug and, if that drug brings relief, to want to repeat its use. Traditionally, the error in viewing addiction within this psychopathology framework has been to selectively emphasize psychopathology as a necessary and sufficient condition to cause addiction, apart from other contributing factors. This has gone hand in hand with strong resistance to seeing the resulting addiction as itself a primary problem in need of specific treatment rather than as a symptom that will be automatically removed once the "real" (psychological) problems are resolved.

Psychological states and dysfunctions that may heighten one's risk of cocaine addiction include depression (the cocaine high produces feelings of pleasure and well-being); other chronic negative mood states, including boredom and fatigue; character disorders such as narcissistic traits (cocaine appeals to the person who seeks self-aggrandizement, because the high is known to induce feelings of powerfulness and confidence); a lack of adequate coping mechanisms (cocaine can provide instant relief from distress and anxiety); and body-image distortions (cocaine decreases appetite, so people who are obsessed with weight tend to be that much more attracted to it). In short, the reinforcing value of cocaine is greater for individuals who exist in a compromised state that could be instantly, though temporarily, improved by cocaine. It is important to remember, however, that while psychological factors can indeed cause or increase one's vulnerability to addictive disease, there is no single personality profile that is common to most cocaine addicts.

Role-modeling

Where one stands on the scale of vulnerability to addictive disease also has to do with certain types of role-modeling one is exposed to, including family role models, peer role models, and societal role models. These factors can converge to cause someone to be highly vulnerable to addiction even if he/she has no preexisting physical predisposition. If a child were to be raised, for example, by a drug-addicted adoptive parent (assuming neither biological parent was chemically dependent) and exposed to pressure from peers to try cocaine, he would probably be high on the vulnerability scale even if free of predisposing physiological vulnerability. Of course, a child raised by a drug-addicted parent would also be likely to suffer from chronic negative mood states and other psychological dysfunctions as a result of growing up in an addictive family.

Access to Cocaine

The other environmental criterion affecting vulnerability is the degree of one's access to the drug. If a person is at high risk for developing addictive disease but never encounters cocaine, then cocaine addiction in particular cannot, of course, occur. That person's addictive disease may express itself in some other ways, such as alcoholism, compulsive gambling, or other addictive and compulsive behaviors. Conversely, those who are frequently exposed to offers of cocaine, because they live in a neighborhood where it is sold on every street corner, for instance, or live in a home where family members make it available, run a high risk of trying cocaine, using it repeatedly, and setting off the addictive disease.

Cocaine Itself

Here we come to the pharmacologic imperatives of cocaine, as described in Chapter 2. The rapid, intense, but very brief cocaine high, the equally unpleasant but prolonged "crash," and the resulting cocaine-induced alterations in brain biochemistry combine to make cocaine the perfect drug for addicting large numbers of users.

Frequency of Use

Related to the dose, method of administration, and pharmacologic effects of cocaine is the frequency of one's use of the drug. Someone who
exposes him/herself to the biochemical action of cocaine once is certainly
not as much at risk of setting the disease in motion as someone who uses it
frequently. In fact, in a person who is otherwise very low on the continuum
of addiction vulnerability, frequent or intensive cocaine use can set off the
addictive response.

The view of cocaine addiction as a disease is undoubtedly gaining acceptance and, as it does so, is transforming the area of treatment. Just as the
addict's cognitive acceptance of addiction as a disease allows him or her to
begin making choices that support recovery, so the treatment field's acceptance of addiction as a disease promotes the design of effective treatment
programs.

CHAPTER 5

Ingredients of Effective Treatment

ALTHOUGH COCAINE ADDICTION is very treatable, no single treatment method is optimal for all cocaine addicts. People who become addicted to cocaine (or anything else, for that matter) are not all the same—they have different needs and different problems. A good deal of judgment and flexibility is required to match the treatment to specific needs of the individual.

The treatment of cocaine addiction has not yet been systematically studied and so no single treatment program or professional discipline can legitimately claim to have the most successful treatment approach. There are, however, some basic guidelines for treating cocaine addicts effectively. Some of these guidelines are similar to those utilized in treating alcoholism and other drug dependencies. The basic task in treating the cocaine addict is to blend what is already known about the effective treatment of chemical dependency in general with techniques and strategies that are specific to cocaine.

In this chapter, we will explore several basic treatment issues, including:

(1) How do you know when cocaine users are addicted to the point of needing treatment?
(2) How do you get cocaine addicts into treatment?
(3) How does the treatment of cocaine addicts differ from the treatment of the alcoholics?

(4) What are the basic ingredients or elements of effective treatment?
(5) When do cocaine addicts require residential care?
(6) When can they be treated entirely on an outpatient basis, without hospitalization?
(7) How can outpatient treatment be made sufficiently intensive to serve as an alternative to residential care?
(8) What is the role of aftercare following residential treatment?

THE NEED FOR TREATMENT

Not everyone who uses cocaine will end up requiring treatment. Some people who use cocaine regularly experience drug-related problems and stop using it on their own — without professional help. Others continue to use the drug despite adverse consequences and find themselves unable to eliminate or drastically reduce their cocaine use despite repeated attempts at restraint and self-control. These are the people who require treatment regardless of their methods of use — snorting, smoking, or injecting cocaine.

The severity of cocaine abuse varies widely among those who seek treatment. The need for treatment is determined not by the method, amount, or frequency of cocaine use, but by the presence of an obsessive involvement with the drug that overshadows other aspects of the person's life and progresses to a point of being beyond the person's volitional control. Many people who fit this description successfully recover from cocaine addiction without formal treatment through personal resolve, a change in life circumstances, and/or involvement in self-help programs such as CA or AA. (Unfortunately, these individuals are not available for scientific study since they do not make contact with any part of the treatment system. Much could be learned from them about why they decided to stop using cocaine, how they did it, and what particular strategies were useful in breaking the habit.) Others either do not want to become involved in self-help programs, preferring to be treated exclusively by professionals, or find that they need a combination of professional treatment and self-help in order to recover successfully.

GETTING THE COCAINE ADDICT INTO TREATMENT

Perhaps the most difficult aspect of treating cocaine addiction is getting the cocaine addict into treatment in the first place. Cocaine addicts rarely seek treatment because they feel that they are using too much cocaine. Attempts to lecture, threaten, plead, or reason with the addict are seldom successful in getting them to seek help. It usually takes a crisis situation or significant personal loss to pierce the addict's wall of denial and motivate him/her to address the problem. For some addicts drug-related consequences must bring them to the brink of personal disaster or serious harm before they even consider the idea of entering treatment. For others, attempts to seek help occur at a much earlier stage of addiction, soon after the negative consequences of chronic drug use cause them significant problems and pain.

The types of problems that most often bring cocaine addicts into treatment involve job, money, and relationships. When faced with the loss of a job or career, inability to pay basic living expenses, or the breakup of a marriage or other valued relationships, the cocaine addict may finally decide to seek help. Some addicts enter treatment because of drug-related legal problems, although this is fairly uncommon among those who are employed. Relatively few cocaine addicts seek treatment because of serious medical problems, although some do show medical problems such as nasal sores or perforations, chest congestion and wheezing, hepatitis, and a history of cocaine-induced convulsions. However, while these problems may lead the cocaine user to seek medical attention at a doctor's office or emergency room for symptomatic relief and reassurance that the problem is not life-threatening, rarely do such problems, in the absence of other drug-related life complications, lead the cocaine user to seek treatment for the addiction.

Unfortunately, no one has yet discovered a reliable way to get addicts to confront the reality of their self-destructive behavior at the earliest stages of drug involvement, before the consequences become too severe. Often concerned others can do very little to stop the addict who is intent on getting high and unwilling to seek help. What they can do, however, is to absolutely and categorically stop "enabling" the addict, that is, stop supporting the addiction and shielding the addict from the negative consequences that naturally follow from dysfunctional, irresponsible, drug-related behavior. (See Chapter 10 for details.)

Family members are often forced into the untenable position of having to stand by, feeling helpless and frustrated, while the addict sends him/herself "down the tubes" into destruction, despair, or even death. For many, this position is totally unacceptable. They feel compelled to do something other than stand by and watch the addict "hit bottom."

Sometimes a group of family members and/or concerned others attempt to "short-circuit" the addict's destructive course. They may decide to collectively confront him/her with the realities of the drug problem and its adverse consequences in a straightforward, nonhostile manner. They may stipulate, for example, that as a prerequisite to receiving any further help from them, the addict must immediately enter a treatment program. In addition to withdrawing their assistance, they may spell out other consequences aimed not at punishing the addict but rather at reducing his/her ability to continue down the path of self-destruction.

This process is sometimes called "raising the bottom," when orchestrated in a more formal way by an addiction treatment professional, it is called an "intervention." It doesn't always work and can be dangerous if not done carefully. Intervention should be considered a last resort, to be used only when other less drastic actions have already failed. Many interventions have saved lives and spared addicts and their families a great deal of unnecessary suffering. But there is always the possibility that the intervention will make things worse by precipitating a suicide attempt or another form of danger-ous acting-out behavior. The need for careful assessment, planning, and professional guidance in the intervention cannot be overemphasized.

Even after the cocaine addict enters treatment there is no guarantee that he/she will actually be receptive to the treatment process. It is not uncom-mon for the addict early in treatment to persistently deny and downplay the severity of the addiction and to resist suggestions aimed at changing lifestyle and behavior. A major part of beginning treatment, therefore, involves increasing the patient's motivation to accept and deal with his/her addiction.

All cocaine addicts who enter treatment are ambivalent about giving up cocaine. When they are in the throes of experiencing negative consequences from their addiction they often want to stop. But once these drug-related crises have passed, the desire for cocaine usually returns. Because the ad-dict's memory of the pain and problems caused by the drug use tends to be short-lived, this alone tends not to supply enough motivation to sustain recovery from cocaine addiction. The required level of motivation must come from the addict's genuine belief in and acceptance of the fact that the problem exists, that there can be no return to occasional drug use without a loss of control and negative consequences, and that recovery will lead to a much improved quality of life.

COCAINE ADDICTION VS. OTHER CHEMICAL DEPENDENCIES

Since the large demand for treatment of cocaine addiction has preceded the development of specialized treatment tracks or programs, many cocaine addicts are currently being treated in general alcoholism and chemical de-pendency programs. Many alcoholism treatment programs, despite a long record of success in treating alcoholics, find cocaine addicts very difficult to treat. Moreover, their success rates with these patients tend to be very poor. This should be no surprise, considering that many of these providers simply have not incorporated into their programs specific treatment components to meet the clinical needs of the cocaine-addicted patient. In some of these programs the problem is one of rigidity—a refusal or inability to see that cocaine addiction differs from alcoholism in ways that require significant adjustments in treatment technique. To these treatment providers, the cocaine addict is seen as an alcoholic who just happened to choose a different drug; consequently, the treatment approach that works for the alcoholic should work for the cocaine addict.

Programs for treating heroin addicts are also having problems treating cocaine addicts, but for somewhat different reasons. Many of these programs have relied on pharmacologic treatment approaches, such as methadone or other substitute drugs, and therefore have never developed expertise in abstinence-oriented treatment. These treatment providers continue to feel "impotent" without some drug or medication upon which the treatment can be based. They tend to get stuck on the cocaine detoxification problem and fail to devise nonpharmacologic treatment strategies for helping cocaine addicts get off and stay off cocaine. Even many of the so-called "drug-free" treatment programs, originally designed to help the already-detoxified heroin addict remain off heroin, have not adequately modified or expanded their services to accommodate the needs of the cocaine addict.

Is treating the cocaine addict really very different from treating the alcoholic? The answer is both yes and no. Treating cocaine addiction probably has more in common with treating alcoholism than with treating any other drug dependency. And there are many more similarities between the two than there are differences—the same basic principles of abstinence-oriented treatment for addictive disease apply equally well to both problems. But the cocaine addict is not simply an alcoholic who just happened to choose a different drug. There are at least several important factors that require adjustments in clinical techniques:

(1) Cocaine and alcohol are pharmacologic opposites. Cocaine is a potent CNS stimulant; alcohol is a potent CNS depressant. Cocaine is often taken to enhance performance and may actually do so during the early "honeymoon" period of use. By contrast, alcohol disrupts brain function and almost always disrupts behavior and performance. Unlike alcohol, cocaine leaves no telltale odor on the user's breath and does not impair motor coordination in a way that would make others aware of the user's intoxication. Except in extreme cases, cocaine use is very difficult to detect on the basis of visual observation alone.

The particular pharmacologic effects of a drug that the user seeks out are not insignificant, incidental, or accidental. People do not take alcohol in order to feel energetic and perform better at work; they do not take cocaine in order to feel relaxed and tranquilized. The clinician should seek to understand the particular "fit" between the person and the drug. What role does drug use play in the individual's life? How has the chosen substance been used to compensate for certain deficits in coping skills or to satisfy unrealistic desires for a "magical solution" to real-life problems?

Since there are basic pharmacologic differences between cocaine and alcohol, cocaine-specific education must be included in the treatment of all cocaine addicts. The education should focus on cocaine first and other drugs second, instead of vice versa.

(2) Cocaine addiction develops and progresses much more rapidly than alcoholism. Alcoholism often develops and progresses over an extremely long period of time, possibly spanning many years. Alcoholics entering treatment may report 10 to 15 years of heavy drinking, with a long list of personal losses and consequences associated with their gradual progression into addictive disease. By contrast, cocaine addiction develops rapidly, sometimes even within a few months after first use. This is especially true with the more intensive routes of administration, such as freebase smoking and IV use. In recounting their history of use, many cocaine addicts are hard-pressed to identify exactly where the problem developed—it seems that all of a sudden they went from controlled use to uncontrolled use with little or no transition period. When cocaine addiction develops very rapidly, it sometimes makes it more difficult for both the user and the family to accept the fact that the problem truly exists, not only because the problem has progressed so quickly, almost before anyone knows what's happening, but also because many of the adverse psychosocial consequences of the compulsive cocaine use have yet to catch up with them.

(3) Cocaine addicts tend to identify best with other cocaine addicts, at least at the beginning of treatment. Just as alcoholics benefit greatly from the presence of role models who are themselves recovering alcoholics, cocaine addicts benefit from having the opportunity for role-modeling and identification with peers successfully recovering from cocaine addiction. This means that wherever possible cocaine addicts should be placed into recovery groups that include at least several other cocaine addicts. In addition, programs treating cocaine addicts should have at least some members of the counseling staff who are themselves recovering cocaine addicts in solid recovery.

However, cocaine addicts should not be segregated into separate treatment programs or separate treatment groups from alcoholics and other chemically dependent patients. Many cocaine addicts already suffer from an exaggerated sense of uniqueness and elitism—they consider themselves to be a "cut above" heroin addicts and alcoholics. It is usually helpful for cocaine addicts to see that their chemical dependency is a variation of addictive disease and not a special problem unto itself.

(4) Cocaine addiction is associated with powerful urges and cravings that dominate the early abstinence period. The beginning phase of treatment

with alcoholics often focuses on detoxification and on regaining normal cognitive functions that were disrupted by chronic alcohol use. While there is no medically dangerous cocaine withdrawal syndrome to manage and no need for substitute drugs to gradually wean the patient from cocaine, abrupt cessation of cocaine use typically brings on powerful cravings and urges which, if not properly handled, lead the patient immediately back to cocaine use. (See Chapter 7 for specific techniques for handling cravings and urges.)

(5) Cocaine is illegal; alcohol is not. As a result, cocaine addicts (especially patients who have both dealt and used illegal drugs) are more often guarded and suspicious toward treatment staff and extremely concerned about issues of confidentiality. These concerns should not be categorically dismissed as cocaine-induced paranoia. Involvement with illegal drugs often engenders deceptive, manipulative, and devious behavior which may not be commonly seen in alcoholics. The treatment professional must be prepared to deal with this type of behavior without being judgmental or personally offended.

BASIC INGREDIENTS OF EFFECTIVE TREATMENT

Although no single treatment method is best for all cocaine addicts, there are at least several basic guidelines for successful treatment. These include the following:

A Structured Treatment Program

In order to successfully recover from cocaine addiction, most addicts will require an addiction treatment program, preferably, one that is highly structured. The necessary level of intensity, structure, accountability, and specific focus on recovery issues is usually offered only in specialized addiction treatment programs. Most cocaine addicts who seek treatment recognize their need for external structure and are often relieved by the clear framework provided by a program that addresses the drug problem directly. Ideally, the rules and expectations of the program regarding abstinence, attendance, etc., will be laid out in writing at the very outset of treatment in an agreement or treatment contract signed by the patient and possibly family members (see Chapter 7). More importantly, the basic rules and guidelines of the program must be implemented fairly and consistently. Failure to set appropriate limits with addicts is a dangerous form of enabling which supports rather than discourages continued drug use. But rigid, irrational limit-setting motivated by a clinician's frustration and annoyance can be even more harmful. It is essential to strike an appropriate balance between firmness and flexibility.

Although most cocaine addicts will require a structured program, some will accept only individual treatment from a private practitioner. While treating cocaine addicts successfully in private practice is certainly possible, it requires a therapist who is skilled and experienced in treating drug addiction and able to offer the appropriate level of treatment structure and intensity, including individual, family, and group counseling, as well as supervised urine testing. Treating the cocaine addict with individual therapy alone, without the support of self-help meetings, group therapy, and family involvement, is often unsuccessful or only temporarily ameliorative.

Because cocaine addicts typically complain of depression, anxiety, and extreme difficulty in relationships, the general psychotherapist (especially one whose approach is psychodynamically oriented) may get "hooked in" to the addict's enabling system by focusing on the multitude of interpersonal and self-esteem problems being generated (or exacerbated) by the drug use. Therapists who are not experienced and skilled in treating drug addiction should be avoided by cocaine addicts, unless they refer the patient to an addiction treatment program and work cooperatively with the program in a joint treatment plan. At least temporarily all attempts at insight-oriented psychotherapy should be put aside in favor of supportive counseling that reinforces the patient's attempt to achieve and maintain abstinence from all mood-altering chemicals.

Treatment in Stages

Recovery from cocaine addiction does not occur all at once or instantaneously—no matter what the treatment approach. Treatment should proceed in a stepwise fashion, in stages where the patient and program focus sequentially on specific tasks and goals, as outlined in Table 5.1.

Although this outline is useful in conceptualizing the treatment and recovery process, there are no rigid dividing lines between the different stages of treatment. In addition, patients may enter at different stages and progress through them at different rates. Nevertheless, dividing treatment into phases is of value not only in defining the basic framework of a treatment program, but also in giving patients a sense of accomplishment and reward as they complete each phase. In terms of total length of treatment, a comprehensive program should require the patient to attend group and individual counseling sessions on a regular basis for a minimum of six months. In most cases six to twelve months is optimal for long-term success.

Absolute Abstinence from Cocaine

Total abstinence from cocaine is the first and foremost goal of beginning treatment. Attempts to cut down rather than stop altogether are rarely successful, since any involvement with cocaine whatsoever is likely to lure

TABLE 5.1
Stages of Treatment

STAGE 1
Stabilization & Crisis Intervention (First 2 Weeks)

Immediately stop all drug and alcohol use
Break off contact with dealers and users
Recover from acute aftereffects and drug "withdrawal"
Stabilize daily functioning
Stabilize or resolve immediate crisis situations
Establish a positive connection to the treatment program
Formulate a treatment plan

STAGE 2
Early Abstinence (Months 1 & 2)

Learn about addictive disease
Admit that the addiction exists
Establish a support system
Begin involvement in self-help
Achieve stable abstinence for at least two weeks

STAGE 3
Relapse Prevention (Months 3 Thru 6)

Progress from verbally admitting to emotionally accepting that the disease exists
Learn about the relapse process, relapse warning signs, relapse risk factors, and how
   to counteract them
Make positive, lasting changes in life-style
Learn how to deal effectively with problems, adjustments, and setbacks
Learn how to identify and handle negative feelings
Learn how to have fun without drugs
Deepen involvement in self-help
Maintain stable abstinence for at least 6 months

STAGE 4
Advanced Recovery (Open-ended)

Achieve more lasting changes in attitude, lifestyle, and behavior
Change addictive thinking styles and personality traits
Address issues of arrested maturity
Solidify adaptive coping and problem-solving skills
Work through emotional, relationship, and self-esteem problems
Continue and deepen involvement in self-help

the addict back into compulsive use. Once the invisible line into addiction is crossed, the ability to return to occasional or "controlled" use is lost forever. Many cocaine addicts enter treatment harboring the hidden intention of resuming occasional use someday—when current pressures to stop all usage subside and the addiction problem is "fixed" by the treatment program. To prevent sabotage of treatment efforts, patients must be educated about this common error in thinking and helped to realize that cocaine addicts never get a second "honeymoon" with cocaine.

Abstinence from Other Psychoactive Drugs

The cocaine addict must give up not only cocaine, but also all other mood-altering addictive drugs. Requiring total abstinence insures the widest margin of safety against potential relapse to cocaine and prevents the development of a substitute addiction. The major goal of recovery is to develop and maintain a reasonably satisfying, productive lifestyle without the use of any mood-altering chemicals. Obviously, this process is stalled while the addict is continuing to use any drugs whatsoever.

Many cocaine addicts who enter treatment strongly object to the idea of giving up all other drugs, especially alcohol and marijuana. "After all," some argue, "I've never had a problem with alcohol or marijuana. I never used them daily, compulsively, or to the point where they interfered with my life. I don't understand why I can't continue to have a single glass of wine or beer with dinner and why I can't smoke a joint once in a while to relax after a hard day at work. I'm not an alcoholic or a 'garbagehead' like some of the other people in this program. My only problem is cocaine. The program's rule of total abstinence is unwarranted and irrational in my case. Why should I stay abstinent from everything?"

The major reasons for insisting on total abstinence as the safest course for recovery from cocaine addiction are as follows:

(a) Other drugs can trigger strong cravings for cocaine. Most cocaine addicts have used other drugs (especially depressants such as alcohol, tranquilizers, sleeping pills, or opiates) to counteract the unpleasant stimulant aftereffects of cocaine or to alleviate the depression and irritability characteristic of the cocaine "crash." By being paired or associated with cocaine literally hundreds or thousands of times, these drugs acquire the ability (through the process of associative conditioning) to elicit powerful urges and cravings for cocaine. They become "reminders" or "triggers" for cocaine in user's brain, setting off a chain reaction that usually starts with drug cravings and ends with drug use. Even patients who have no history of alcohol abuse prior to cocaine addiction may find that a single glass of beer or wine sets off irresistible cravings for cocaine.

(b) Getting high on any drug inevitably puts the cocaine addict one step closer to cocaine. Most mood-altering drugs have a "disinhibiting" effect on the user's attitude and behavior; that is, when high on *any* drug most people tend to feel "looser" and more likely to act on their impulses. Thus, the use of any mood-altering drug is likely to render the abstaining cocaine addict more vulnerable to offers of cocaine or to acting on an impulse for cocaine.

(c) Other drugs provide substitute highs which can lead to substitute addictions. When deprived of their drug of choice, cocaine addicts often find other drugs more appealing for substitute highs. This is especially true for alcohol, because it is often the only "legitimate" way left for the abstaining cocaine addict to get inconspicuously high. Alcohol is legal, readily available, and often socially encouraged even by family members and friends who make the mistake of thinking that the cocaine addict's problem is limited only to cocaine.

While abstaining from cocaine, the user may develop other drug dependencies, complicating and stalling the recovery process. In cases where the cocaine addict has a history of other drug dependencies before cocaine addiction, the use of any mood-altering drug is likely to rekindle these problems. Some patients deny their previous addictions while others may purposely keep this information hidden from their therapist or peers in order to better rationalize the safety of their continued use.

(d) Other drugs may prevent the biochemical recovery of brain functioning disrupted by cocaine. Most mood-altering drugs have diffuse and overlapping effects on neurotransmitter systems and other biochemical functions in the brain. Thus, any drug use whatsoever may impede the natural healing process by which the brain's homeostatic mechanisms seek to reverse the neurological insult caused by chronic cocaine use. Total abstinence provides the widest margin of safety in terms of allowing maximal physiological recovery of brain function in the shortest period of time. It remains to be seen whether the neurological disruption caused by cocaine is partially or totally reversible with complete abstinence.

Education

Treatment should include a strong educational component to provide the patient with a basic framework for understanding his/her addiction in a way that facilitates the treatment and recovery process. Education can be a very powerful treatment tool for bringing about changes in attitude and behavior and actively involving the patient in his/her own treatment. Family members should receive education as well. Topics covered in education sessions should include the basic pharmacology and effects of cocaine and other addictive drugs, basic principles of addictive disease and recovery, early warning signs of relapse and how to prevent relapses from occurring, an introduction to self-help programs, the family dynamics of addiction, enabling and co-dependency, and an overview of medical and psychosocial consequences of addiction.

Family Involvement

Chemical dependency is almost always a family disease in terms of its etiology, maintenance, and negative impact. In many cases, recovery of the cocaine addict is extraordinarily difficult or impossible without the participation of key family members. In addition to supplying useful information that confirms, refutes, or elaborates upon the patient's report, family members are often themselves sorely in need of advice and guidance on how to deal with the addict's manipulative and exploitive behavior. They sometimes contribute to the perpetuation of the addiction with enabling and supporting behaviors: (a) giving the addict money that goes directly or indirectly to drugs; (b) making excuses to others for the addict's irresponsible behavior; (c) doing other things to shield the addict from the negative consequences of his/her drug use; and (d) acting out their own anger and feelings of helplessness on the addict in a way that allows the addict to conveniently blame family members rather than taking personal responsibility for the problems in his/her life. Not only must family members learn how to help the addict more constructively, but they must also be helped to find more adaptive ways to deal with the justifiable feelings of anger, frustration, helplessness, and sadness stemming from their futile attempts to "fix" the addict's problem (see Chapter 10).

Urine Testing

Requiring the patient to give a supervised urine sample at frequent intervals enables the clinician to reliably detect the use of any drugs or to verify abstinence. The purpose of urine testing is not to catch the addict in a lie, but rather to help him/her exert better control over impulses to use drugs by establishing accountability. This often helps to break through the denial and self-deceit that is characteristic of addictive disease and contributes to continuing drug use. Simply knowing that any drug use will be detected in the urine may enable the patient to resist temptation in an otherwise difficult situation. This is probably why most drug addicts who enter treatment are relieved rather than offended by the requirement of urine testing. If a program requires urine testing, patients know that they will not be able to relapse without being noticed — a comforting fact to most, despite their continuing ambivalence about giving up cocaine.

One patient observed: "As far as urine testing goes, my first reaction was shock and outrage. On second thought, however, I was delighted to know that there was a backstop. I'd have to go through a lot of scheming to have a relapse and hide it from the program. I'm glad it's there. It's another tool that's helping me to stay clean."

In addition to serving as a built-in safety mechanism, urine testing prevents patients from devaluing a therapist or program whom they have been able to deceive and manipulate and provides them with a concrete measure of treatment progress. In fact, patients often ask to see the lab reports verifying that their urine is "clean." Family members often breathe a little easier knowing that the addict is on a schedule of urine surveillance. They can give up their attempts to guess "did he or didn't he?" and to observe even the slightest behavioral signs that the addict may have used drugs again.

In order for urine testing to be of maximum clinical value, these procedural guidelines should be followed:

(1) All samples should be witnessed (observed) in order to prevent falsification, samples "brought in" by patients should never be accepted.
(2) A sample should be collected at least every three to four days so as not to exceed the sensitivity of laboratory detection methods for most drugs.
(3) Testing should be done by enzyme-immunoassay or radio-immunoassay procedures to insure accuracy. Less expensive tests such as thin layer chromatography (TLC) are not accurate enough for short-acting drugs like cocaine.
(4) Urine testing procedures should be continued throughout the entire course of treatment. Patients should not be given the message that they will "graduate" from urine testing.

Group and Individual Therapy

A combination of group and individual therapy is optimal in most cases. Group therapy is the core of most treatment approaches for addicts — and cocaine addicts are no exception. A recovery group comprised of cocaine addicts and other chemically dependent persons provides an opportunity to identify with peers, receive group support and reassurance, learn about addiction and recovery, and confront maladaptive attitudes and behaviors. In individual therapy specific individual issues, such as psychological, sexual, and interpersonal problems that may have existed before the addiction or developed as a result of it, can be addressed.

Self-help Groups

Cocaine addicts should be strongly encouraged to become involved in the 12-step program of Cocaine Anonymous (CA), Narcotics Anonymous (NA), or Alcoholics Anonymous (AA). Exposure to these self-help programs should be routinely provided by all professional treatment programs. Self-help meetings offer an invaluable source of support and assistance at no cost (see Chapter 9).

Alternative Activities

Physical exercise, sports, and other recreational activities are an important part of building a healthier lifestyle, which will in turn support a lasting recovery from cocaine addiction. Physical activity can relieve stress, improve mood, and instill positive feelings of having greater control over one's life.

Nutritional, Medical, and Dental Care

Neglect of one's physical health and general well-being is common among cocaine addicts. Many have lost weight, ignored chronic medical problems, and perpetuated or intensified poor eating habits. A comprehensive medical, dental, and nutritional evaluation is indicated in most cases, followed by proper treatment and counseling.

Pharmacologic Therapy

A "magic bullet" to cure cocaine addiction will probably never be found, but cocaine addicts who truly have coexisting psychiatric disorders that may be responsive to nonaddictive therapeutic medications should certainly not be deprived of those medications simply because they are drug addicts. The indications for using psychotropic medications in cocaine addicts are identical to those in individuals who suffer from the same psychiatric disorders but are not addicts—the only major exception being that drug addicts and alcoholics should never be given psychotropic medications that have an acute mood-altering effect, since all such drugs are potentially addictive.

INPATIENT VS. OUTPATIENT CARE

Outpatient treatment is preferable to inpatient (residential) care whenever the clinical status and life circumstances of the patient allow it. Therefore, one of the first decisions to be made in treating the cocaine addict is whether he/she can be treated entirely on an outpatient basis or will first require inpatient care in a hospital or residential drug rehabilitation facility. Since cocaine does not produce an acute withdrawal syndrome that jeopardizes physical health or requires medical management, few medical reasons for requiring addicts to be treated in an inpatient setting exist.

Advantages of Outpatient Care

There are at least several distinct advantages to outpatient treatment over inpatient treatment, including:

(1) It is less expensive, less disruptive to the addict's work and home life, and less stigmatizing.

(2) It is usually more acceptable to the addict; sometimes it is the only form of treatment the cocaine addict will accept. Refused the option of ambulatory treatment, many cocaine addicts flatly refuse to enter treatment at all — perpetuating their addiction and causing further damage to themselves and others. Thus, the option of outpatient treatment reduces some of the obstacles that keep cocaine addicts from entering treatment in the first place.

(3) Outpatient treatment has certain clinical advantages. While inpatient treatment temporarily removes the cocaine addict from ready access to drugs, it may not adequately prepare the patient for remaining abstinent after hospital discharge — as evidenced by the fact that relapse rates after inpatient treatment remain extraordinarily high. Outpatient treatment teaches the cocaine addict to manage his/her drug compulsion within the "real world" rather than the artificially safe environment of an inpatient facility. Treatment can focus immediately on the inevitable task of learning how to manage daily life without drugs — despite the availability of cocaine and the presence of environmental cues that trigger cocaine cravings.

No studies to date have produced convincing evidence that treatment in residential settings is more effective than outpatient treatment. On the contrary, studies show either no significant differences between treatment settings or differences favoring outpatient treatment.

Despite its potential advantages, outpatient treatment for cocaine addiction (and other chemical dependencies) remains grossly underutilized. This picture is changing, however — especially with the current trend toward developing more cost-effective treatment approaches and the resulting emergence of a new treatment modality, namely, the intensive outpatient rehabilitation program. This treatment approach provides a level of clinical care that closely approximates inpatient treatment, but at a much lower cost and without disruption to the patient's work and home life.

With the increasing nationwide emphasis on containing health care costs and the unprecedented rates at which drug addicts have been entering treatment (due largely to the cocaine epidemic), more attention is being paid to the development of cost-effective outpatient treatment models. The impetus is coming in large part from employers and from other third-party payers, such as health insurance companies and prepaid health plans which continue to foot the enormous bills for sending drug addicts to hospitals and inpatient rehabilitation centers—where a single 30-day treatment episode can cost anywhere from $5,000 to $35,000.

As more consumers of addiction treatment and employers realize that residential treatment is simply not required in most cases, outpatient treatment will become the treatment of choice. Few addicts want to leave their home and job in order to receive treatment—unless it is absolutely required. Employers, too, would rather not pull someone off the job—causing a loss in productivity, disruption of ongoing projects, the extra cost of replacement labor, and a big hospital rehabilitation bill—if instead the employee can remain on the job while being treated effectively in an outpatient program. If designed properly, an intensive outpatient rehabilitation program can combine the structure and intensity of an inpatient program with the convenience, acceptability, and cost-effectiveness of an outpatient program.

Intensive Outpatient Treatment

Let's take a brief look at the elements of an intensive outpatient rehabilitation program. Since this is the major modality of treatment offered at The Washton Institute, I will use my program as an example. The program lasts for a total of six months, with an optional continuing care component for an additional six months. The six-month program is divided into two phases—the intensive outpatient rehabilitation program, which lasts two months, and the relapse prevention program, which lasts four months. The goal of the intensive program is to help the active drug user break the cycle of addiction, establish early abstinence from all mood-altering chemicals, and initiate positive changes in attitude, lifestyle, and behavior. Patients attend group therapy sessions, educational lectures, and self-help meetings four evenings per week, usually for at least three hours each evening. In addition, they receive individual, marital, and family counseling at least once per week. Family members attend an eight-week family education and counseling program, meeting once a week, to help them deal with enabling behavior and other co-dependency problems.

Upon completing the intensive program, patients enter the relapse prevention program, which concentrates on maintaining abstinence, avoiding relapse, and learning how to deal effectively with problems and adjustments through the first six months of recovery. Patients attend group therapy sessions, educational lectures, and self-help meetings three evenings per week and also receive individual and/or marital/family counseling once per week. Family members attend an ongoing family recovery group, with separate groups for spouses and parents.

Thus far, over 80 percent of patients admitted to the program have successfully completed it and we are now in the process of collecting follow-up data to evaluate long-term success rates. Prior to implementing the intensive program, we found it necessary to refer at least 35 percent of all treatment applicants to residential care. Now fewer than 15 percent of our applicants require inpatient treatment. In other words, utilization of inpatient treatment has been cut by more than 50 percent — with no apparent compromise in the quality or effectiveness of patient care. Preliminary data suggest that our program may be capable of producing substantially higher long-term success rates than traditional inpatient care.

Inpatient Treatment

Despite the advantages of intensive outpatient treatment, some cocaine addicts will nonetheless require residential care. An inpatient setting offers certain advantages that an outpatient program cannot — especially when the cocaine addict is severely dysfunctional, debilitated, or suffering from serious medical and psychiatric complications. Inpatient treatment immediately halts the drug use, removes the cocaine addict from a destructive lifestyle, and prevents access to drugs. Especially when cocaine use is accompanied by extremely dangerous or self-destructive behavior, such as suicide attempts, violence, or other types of acting-out behavior with potentially severe, life-damaging consequences, residential treatment is imperative. In such cases, residential treatment may indeed be life-saving and offers the safest place for treatment to begin.

Inpatient treatment may also be needed when attempts at outpatient treatment have failed or when the cocaine addict's psychiatric status and level of functioning have deteriorated to the point where outpatient treatment is highly risky or impossible. The major clinical indications for inpatient treatment of the cocaine addict are:

(1) The cocaine addict is suicidal, violent, psychotic, or otherwise dangerous to him/herself or others.

(2) The cocaine addict has severe medical and/or psychiatric problems requiring intensive observation and/or treatment.
(3) The cocaine addict is so dysfunctional that he/she is unable to manage the basic tasks of daily living.
(4) The cocaine addict is physically dependent on alcohol and/or drugs (other than cocaine) requiring detoxification and close medical supervision in an inpatient setting.
(5) The cocaine addict is unable to comply with or fails to benefit sufficiently from an outpatient treatment program.

Inpatient treatment, when required, must be seen as only the first step or "launching pad" in recovery from cocaine addiction. The major goals of inpatient treatment should be to break the cycle of compulsive drug use, stabilize the patient's functioning, and strengthen the patient's motivation for continued treatment following hospital discharge.

"Aftercare" Treatment

The term "aftercare" seems to connote that outpatient treatment following residential care is merely an "afterthought," when actually the most critical phase of recovery begins after the addict leaves the protection of the hospital environment and enters outpatient treatment. It is extremely unlikely that completion of an inpatient treatment program, by itself, will ever produce lifelong abstinence and recovery from cocaine addiction. Relapse rates following inpatient treatment remain extraordinarily high for cocaine addicts who do not continue their treatment in a structured and intensive outpatient program for at least several months following residential care.

CHAPTER 6

Assessment

A THOROUGH CLINICAL assessment of the cocaine addict is the starting point of all good treatment. The initial interview is a critical event—one that often determines whether the cocaine addict accepts treatment at all, and if so, with what degree of optimism and cooperation. Among the major goals of the assessment are: (1) to establish a beginning therapeutic alliance with the patient; (2) to gather the relevant clinical data in order to formulate an initial treatment plan that specifically addresses the patient's individual needs; and (3) to orient the patient to the procedures, requirements, and expectations of the treatment program.

WHO IS BEING EVALUATED?

Although it is ostensibly the patient who is being evaluated, the initial interview is always a two-way evaluation. Both the patient and the clinician give and receive information about one another that leads to the formation of initial impressions and conclusions by both parties. Addicts can usually "size up" strangers very quickly (a skill with obvious adaptive value for those using illegal drugs). During the interview, most are acutely aware of the clinician's body language, facial expressions, tone of voice, and choice of words. Among the many questions and concerns that the applicant may have about the clinician (whether verbalized or not) are the following:

- Does this person have a sophisticated understanding of drugs — especially of cocaine, cocaine use, and cocaine addiction?
- Does this person have a judgmental or negative attitude about addicts?
- Is this person willing to invest the time and effort to understand me as an individual — or does he/she operate according to preconceived, fixed ideas about addicts and their problems?
- Is this someone whom I can trust with confidential information?
- Is this someone who really knows how to help me with my cocaine problem?
- What is this person's view of addiction and its treatment?
- Is this person knowledgeable and competent?
- Is this person compassionate and human?
- Can I count on this person for both firmness and understanding?
- Is this person a self-confident, "take charge" type of individual whom I can rely on for support and guidance when things get rough?
- How easily can I con and manipulate this person?
- Is this person interested in me or primarily in the money?
- Will this person be available when I need him/her?
- What is this person's record of success in treating cocaine addicts?

Clearly, the initial interview is much more than just a formal history-taking or fact-gathering procedure. It is quite literally the beginning of treatment. It is at this point that the all-important process of establishing a good working alliance with the patient begins. The strength of the patient's early connection to the interviewer should not be underestimated. Later in treatment patients often refer to this first contact, saying how relieved they felt at being listened to and understood by someone who was nonjudgmental and able to describe a clear, rational approach to dealing with their problem when everything felt hopeless and bleak. The beginning therapeutic contact with the patient can go a long way toward fostering a receptive, cooperative attitude that enhances the treatment and recovery process.

ASSESSMENT PROCEDURES

The initial interview supplies the information needed to formulate a temporary treatment plan for at least the first week or so of the patient's treatment. However, the assessment of a treatment applicant is an ongoing process that continues indefinitely as an integral part of treatment; it cannot and should not be completed within a single interview or visit. Information gathered during the initial interview is often supplemented and modified during the course of subsequent contact with the patient in ways that may dictate significant changes in treatment strategies. For example, the patient may subsequently divulge that he/she is in the midst of a severe marital, legal, medical, or financial crisis which necessitates more frequent visits, involvement of a spouse or other family members in the treatment, or coordination of the treatment with other professionals.

The initial assessment should cover a wide range of issues, including:

(1) the current reasons and motivation for seeking treatment;
(2) the current severity of cocaine use, with a detailed description of the pattern, frequency, amount, chronicity, circumstances, and method/route of administration;
(3) a similarly detailed description of current use of alcohol and any other mood-altering drugs;
(4) the presence and severity of drug-related medical and psychosocial problems;
(5) the history of previous drug/alcohol use and the progression from initial use to regular use and addiction;
(6) a detailed description of previous periods of abstinence and/or treatment attempts, including the dates and length of these periods as well as the circumstances and precipitants of relapse;
(7) the presence and severity of nonchemical addictions, including compulsive gambling, compulsive sexuality, eating disorders, etc., and any previous treatment for these problems;
(8) a detailed psychiatric history and assessment of current psychiatric status;
(9) a detailed family history, including the presence of psychiatric illness and substance abuse problems in immediate family members;
(10) the nature of current relationships with family members and the existing family support structure;
(11) educational and occupational history, including any current indebtedness and involvement in drug dealing;
(12) current and pending legal status;
(13) current mental status — (keep in mind that a valid assessment interview cannot be conducted when the patient is actively intoxicated or "crashing" from cocaine and/or other drugs); and
(14) the patient's expectations of treatment, desire for change, and current beliefs about the nature and severity of his/her drug problem and what type of assistance would be most helpful.

To facilitate the process of evaluating treatment applicants, I developed several years ago a detailed assessment questionnaire—the Cocaine Assessment Profile or CAP (see Appendix A)—a self-administered intake form that the treatment applicant fills out in the waiting room immediately prior to the initial interview. Another assessment tool, a 38-item rating scale—the Cocaine Addiction Severity Test or CAST (Appendix B)—provides a rough measure of the severity of the patient's cocaine addiction problem. Few, if any, cocaine users in need of treatment will score less than 10 on this rating scale. Those who score above 30 will generally require the most intensive efforts to achieve abstinence as outpatients, and some may need residential care before being able to benefit from an outpatient program.

Use of the CAP and CAST thus far with over 1,500 primary cocaine addicts indicates that these simple, self-administered evaluation tools not only save time, but also serve a therapeutic function. Filling out these questionnaires often heightens the applicant's awareness of just how serious his/her drug problem really is and how badly it is damaging his/her life. This is usually the first time that the applicant has been asked to provide a detailed account of his/her drug use and its resulting consequences—an experience that often helps to pierce the addict's denial system.

Another benefit of using a self-administered questionnaire is that it frees the clinician from spending his/her first contact with the patient busily writing down historical information, instead the session can be devoted primarily to acquiring a beginning understanding of the applicant and his/her problem and to interacting more directly with the applicant in a way that sets the stage for effective treatment.

Reasons for Seeking Treatment

The specific reasons why the cocaine addict has decided to seek treatment and why he/she is doing it now rather than last week or last month are among the most important early issues to be addressed. It is essential to find out specifically what drug-related problem is causing the applicant the most distress. Is it a marital problem, a job problem, a financial problem, or some combination of these? This information may provide the key to sustaining the patient's motivation through the early phase of treatment, enabling the clinician to pinpoint areas of difficulty and establish a hierarchy of problems to be addressed. It may also identify motivational problems, as in the case of an applicant who comes to the interview at the behest of someone else and has little or no intention of stopping his/her use of cocaine. Did the applicant agree to talk to a treatment professional just to pacify an irate family member or employer? Is he/she trying to "buy some time" to avoid a threatened consequence? Is there evidence of a genuine internal desire or motivation for treatment? If not, can the applicant be helped to identify some important reasons to stop using cocaine?

Hidden intentions to quickly enter and leave treatment as soon as an immediate crisis is resolved should be brought out in the open through nonjudgmental, nonconfrontational questioning. Gently chipping away at the addict's ambivalence about giving up cocaine may offer the only hope of preventing premature dropout in someone who really does not want to be in treatment in the first place.

Even those who do leave prematurely may benefit later from this attempt to address their ambivalence and denial. Helping the active cocaine addict to see that he/she is actively choosing to reject professional assistance in favor of continuing his/her destructive use of cocaine should not be considered a therapeutic failure, but a first step. This experience may make it easier for the addict to choose treatment at a later time when his/her denial system is more forcefully challenged by an escalation of drug-related consequences. When faced by a cocaine addict who is simply unwilling to accept help, the clinician can, rather than acting out feelings of frustration and helplessness, use this opportunity to educate the applicant about addictive disease and its most insidious symptom — denial.

FEELINGS ABOUT ENTERING TREATMENT

Until the arrival of crack, which made cocaine accessible to just about everyone, cocaine addicts seeking treatment tended to be mainly from middle-class and upper-middle-class backgrounds and were fairly well-functioning. Their history of good functioning, in many cases coupled with the use of marijuana and/or alcohol which never got out of control, led them to believe that they were invulnerable to addiction. When they began using cocaine they appeared, at least on the surface, to be in control of their lives. They had maintained busy work schedules, earned decent incomes, had families and no history of psychiatric problems. Even though most were aware that cocaine could be addictive, they tended to believe that their own self-will and determination (which had helped them to accomplish other tasks) would protect them form succumbing to drug dependency.

For this type of person, needing treatment for drug addiction is experienced as an especially severe personal defeat, running counter to a previously well-maintained self-image of competence, success, and invulnerability — an image often fed by the cocaine high itself. These applicants tend to have strong concerns about confidentiality and greatly fear the stigma that they feel is attached to needing professional help to resolve a personal problem. This subgroup of cocaine addicts can best be reached by helping them to reframe their choice to seek help as a sign of strength and determination — not weakness and defeat. The paradoxical truth is that the addict must admit powerlessness over cocaine in order to regain control over his/her life, an idea that must be introduced early in treatment.

A powerful but often overlooked determinant of prognosis is the patient's own expectations of treatment. Applicants may have unrealistic hopes that treatment will instantly cure them of unmanageable life problems and restore their ability to use cocaine in a controlled way. These common but dangerous fantasies must be addressed at some point during the assessment, where education about addictive disease and recovery begins.

History and Pattern of Cocaine Use

METHOD OF USE

The patient's preferred and current method of administering cocaine is an important clue to the severity of addiction. In general, addiction develops more rapidly and is often more severe in freebase/crack smokers and intravenous users than among snorters (intranasal users). Because smoking cocaine produces more intense drug effects, the user is driven more rapidly toward compulsive patterns of use and consumption of larger quantities of cocaine. Freebase/crack smokers tend also to use other drugs in larger quantities in order to counteract the extremely negative aftereffects of high-dose cocaine use. Freebase/crack and IV users typically report a faster progression from initial to compulsive/addictive use and experience more severe drug-related dysfunction.

However, the addict's method of cocaine administration is not always indicative of addiction severity. A severe addiction can develop with any route of administration, including intranasal use. Cocaine snorters can get just as addicted as freebasers; it just takes them longer.

DOSE

The amount of cocaine that the applicant is regularly consuming provides another measure of addiction severity. How many grams does he/she consume typically in a week? How many grams per day or per episode of use? There is no specific formula or easy equation here for determining exactly how much cocaine use is indicative of abuse or addiction, but in general the more cocaine the applicant is using, the more difficult it will be for him/her to break the cycle of compulsive drug use.

FREQUENCY

Related to dose is the frequency of cocaine use, and this also varies widely in treatment applicants, even among those showing similar levels of drug-induced problems. Frequency of cocaine use can range from sporadic concentrated binges, separated by days or even weeks of temporary abstinence, to continuous use every single day. Although generally speaking, more chronic and more frequent use means more severe addiction, quite often weekend-only and other sporadic users also lose control over their drug intake, become preoccupied with thoughts about cocaine, and suffer negative effects on their health and functioning. While they may not use cocaine every day, they are undoubtedly addicted.

Since binge use rather than daily use is a pattern more common among cocaine users than among other drug abusers, the clinician should be careful not to underestimate the severity of an applicant's addiction simply because he/she boasts of having not used any cocaine for a week or more before the interview. A pattern of high-dose binges separated by several days or weeks of abstinence typically results in problems just as severe, if not more so, than daily usage of much lower doses.

SETTINGS AND CIRCUMSTANCES

A detailed account of the specific settings and circumstances of the patient's cocaine use (e.g., time of day, where, and with whom it is used) helps to identify potential relapse "triggers." For instance, some addicts will use only in the evening or on weekends and associate cocaine with "unwinding" from a hard day's work or with having a good time (using cocaine is often called "partying" whether at a party of not). Others are more likely to use cocaine at work, initially for its performance-enhancing effects, especially in work environments where cocaine use is accepted or even encouraged. It is important to know the answers to the following questions: Does the patient use with a particular friend, family member, or coworker, or mostly when home alone? How and where are drug supplies obtained? Are there constant temptations to use cocaine at home because other members of the household are cocaine users or dealers? This information is useful in helping the patient plan strategies to establish early abstinence.

EXPENSE

Another measure of cocaine consumption is the amount of money the addict is spending on the drug in a typical week or month. This measure, because it is subject to variations in the street price of cocaine and the patient's sources, may reveal less about the amount consumed than about the comparative value of cocaine to the user. Does the patient sell cocaine to offset the cost of his/her own use? What percentage of the patient's salary or income is spent on drugs? Are there depleted bank accounts, overdue bills, accumulating debts on credit cards, and personal loans, all due to cocaine use? Denial can be extremely severe when the cocaine addict's current level of drug use is not causing financial problems or forcing a change in his/her standard of living. For those capable of supporting their drug habit without financial consequence, evidence of adverse effects must be identified in other areas of functioning.

Other Drug Use

Alcohol, marijuana, tranquilizers, sleeping pills, and opiates may be used in substantial amounts by cocaine addicts to counteract or alleviate the unpleasant aftereffects of cocaine, such as anxiety, restlessness, and insomnia. It is common for cocaine addicts to have acquired dependencies on one or more of these drugs without being fully aware of it. Many tend not to appreciate the severity of this other drug use, thinking of it as merely an antidote for the cocaine "jitters." This failure to recognize the problem also stems from the fact that someone under the influence of cocaine can usually consume a fairly hefty dose of depressants (such as alcohol or sedative-hypnotics) without experiencing the typical signs of depressant intoxication, such as slurred speech, stumbling gait, and drowsiness, since the depressant effects on the brain are partially blocked or counteracted by the stimulant effects of the cocaine.

Two critical treatment issues emerge relative to an applicant's other drug use. The first is the importance of insisting on abstinence from these drugs (discussed in Chapter 5). The second is its bearing on whether the applicant will need to be hospitalized for a medically supervised detoxification. Withdrawal from physical dependency on barbiturates, benzodiazepines, or alcohol generally requires the close medical supervision of an inpatient setting to insure maximum safety and comfort. If patients taking these drugs discontinue them too abruptly, they may experience severe withdrawal reactions with potentially serious medical consequences. Withdrawal from heroin and other opiates is not life-threatening, but often the onset of severe withdrawal discomfort makes opiate detoxification difficult to complete successfully on an outpatient basis. Consequently, it is usually easier for the patient to complete this procedure in a hospital.

Other Compulsive Behaviors

Because many cocaine addicts exhibit coexisting problems with other addictive/compulsive behaviors (including sexual addictions, compulsive gambling, and eating disorders), evaluation for the presence of these problems should be routinely included in the assessment procedure. Coexisting but undiagnosed and untreated addictions may increase during treatment or actively precipitate relapse to cocaine.

There are at least a couple of reasons why cocaine addiction is sometimes accompanied by one or more of these other addictions. First, the presence of any addictive disorder may indicate that the person has a propensity to engage in other compulsive mood-altering experiences. This propensity may find expression both through chemicals—and does so particularly when these chemicals are readily accessible—and through compulsively engaging in other kinds of nonchemical activities. Second, cocaine use may be accompanied by (or sometimes facilitate) sexual behavior and gambling, which then become paired with cocaine through the process of associative conditioning. Similarly, cocaine's appetite-suppressing effects are appealing to many compulsive overeaters, bulimics, and anorexics, who find it to be an instant (but temporary and destructive) "cure" for their eating disorders.

COMPULSIVE SEXUALITY

Among cocaine addicts who apply for treatment, some have problems with compulsive sexuality. This is especially true among male freebase smokers. The coexistence of cocaine addiction and compulsive sexuality often creates an insidious, vicious cycle in which the drug use and the sexual behavior reciprocally spark and intensify one another. During periods of attempted abstinence from both addictions, relapse to one almost invariably precipitates relapse to the other.

For example, a 38-year-old male freebase addict reported a compulsive pattern of marathon cocaine smoking binges which involved multiple sexual encounters with prostitutes. These marathon cocaine and sex binges ran continuously from late Friday afternoon to early Monday morning nearly every week. During the first few months of cocaine abstinence, this patient found that even a fleeting sexual thought or fantasy would set off powerful cravings for cocaine as a result of the strong connection between the two. In the course of describing the problem, he said:

> "For me the difficult part of staying off cocaine is the sexual aspect of it. As soon as I start remembering the exotic and erotic experiences I've had while high on cocaine, I start to crave the whole scene again—the girls and the coke. It's extremely difficult for me to separate them—as soon as I get a sexual urge, I immediately think 'cocaine.'"

Another adult male freebase addict reported problems with cocaine and compulsive masturbation. While high on cocaine, he would compulsively masturbate, alone in his apartment, for five or six hours at a time while viewing pornographic videos or magazines and sometimes while dressed up in women's lingerie (which heightened the intensity of his orgasms). These cocaine and sex binges had led him to be fired from at least two jobs because of lateness and absenteeism. Cocaine use fueled his sexual compulsion, but just as importantly, his sexual compulsion fueled his cocaine use. The sexual addiction predated his first use of cocaine by at least several years, but the severity of the sexual problem increased dramatically as soon as he started using cocaine, due to the drug's initial aphrodisiac effects.

These case examples illustrate the powerful, reciprocal effects that can exist between cocaine and sexual addictions. Cocaine can markedly intensify a preexisting sexual compulsion; similarly, a preexisting sexual compulsion can markedly intensify the use of cocaine and speed up the individual's progression into addictive disease. A list of diagnostic questions for determining the presence of sexual addiction/compulsion is presented in Appendix C.

COMPULSIVE GAMBLING

Another addiction prevalent among cocaine addicts is compulsive gambling. Cocaine may fit right in with compulsive gambling because it provides a similar type of stimulant high and illusion of power and success. An addict suffering from chronic boredom or depression may find the highs from gambling and cocaine similarly attractive. Also, cocaine's powerful stimulant effects may enable the compulsive gambler to stay awake energetically for long periods of time while engaging in marathon gambling binges.

The three major diagnostic criteria of compulsive gambling listed in *DSM-III* are: (1) a chronic and progressive inability to resist the urge to gamble; (2) interference with functioning, manifested in at least three of seven areas (family, work, legal, defaulting on debts, borrowing from illegal sources, inability to account for winnings, need for "bailouts"); (3) presence of these signs in the absence of a global antisocial personality disorder.

Because cocaine addiction and compulsive gambling coexist in a significant minority of cocaine addicts seeking treatment, an evaluation of gambling behavior should be routinely included in the clinical assessment procedure. Useful screening instruments are the South Oaks Gambling Screen (SOGS), developed by Lesieur and Blume (see Appendix D), and a questionnaire used at The Washton Institute (Appendix E).

If gambling and cocaine have been paired, then being in a gambling situation in early recovery can easily trigger cocaine cravings and precipitate a relapse. Or, when a patient with a gambling problem becomes abstinent from cocaine, he/she may escalate gambling activity. For these reasons complete abstinence from gambling is usually necessary in any cocaine addict with a history of gambling problems.

COMPULSIVE EATING AND NON-EATING

Among cocaine-addicted women, some have long-standing, fairly severe problems with compulsive overeating, bulimia, and, to a lesser extent, anorexia. They originally use cocaine to control their appetite and initiate or maintain weight loss, but eventually the drug takes control of their lives and they continue using it despite the development of tolerance to its appetite-suppressing benefits. Most of these individuals are obsessed with food and even more obsessed with their body weight and appearance. During early abstinence from cocaine, the slightest weight gain and/or return of normal eating habits may create intense anxiety and fears and trigger a relapse to the drug. These patterns can be revealed only by a careful, detailed assessment of each treatment applicant's eating patterns and their relationship to past or current cocaine use. A sample eating disorders questionnaire is provided in Appendix F.

Life Events

Often escalating cocaine use parallels or follows particular life crises or events. A careful history commonly reveals that events such as divorce, job loss, financial problems, career crises, serious physical or mental illness, death of a loved one, etc. precipitated or otherwise contributed to attempts at chemical coping and escape.

Previous Treatment for Drug or Alcohol Abuse

The current treatment attempt must be placed in the context of the patient's overall "recovery career." What, if any, previous attempts have been made in treatment? Where? When? What type of treatment? How long did the patient stay in treatment and why did he/she leave treatment? Has he or she ever attended Cocaine Anonymous, Alcoholics Anonymous, Narcotics Anonymous, or any other self-help group? What did the patient find helpful about treatment and/or self-help? What was not helpful? What could be done differently this time to increase the chances for success? What gains were made in previous treatments and how long did they last? To what extent does the patient take personal responsibility for previous treatment failure(s), instead of blaming others or the program?

Cocaine-Related Consequences

Careful assessment of the applicant's functioning and identification of drug-related problems or dysfunction are essential to the formulation of an individualized treatment plan. The CAP contains several checklists which cover cocaine-related medical and psychosocial consequences. This information is essential both to evaluating a patient's treatment needs and, as mentioned earlier, to heightening the patient's own awareness of the negative impact cocaine has had on his or her life — a further challenge to denial.

HEALTH PROBLEMS

Although the incidence of serious medical problems in cocaine addicts is fairly low, it is advisable to include a complete physical examination with blood tests, urine tests, and EKG as part of the evaluation procedure. The most commonly expected physical complaints include insomnia, weight loss, anergia, headaches, and sexual dysfunction. Other symptoms vary with the route of administration. Snorters often complain of nasal sores, nasal bleeding, and congested sinuses. Freebase smokers report chest congestion, wheezing, chronic cough, black phlegm, sore throat, and hoarseness. Intravenous users may show abscesses at injection sites, elevated liver enzymes, and systemic infections such as hepatitis and endocarditis. Freebase and IV users also commonly report histories of cocaine-induced brain seizures with loss of consciousness, the result of large drug doses rapidly reaching the brain.

PSYCHOSOCIAL DYSFUNCTION

Generally, the more severe the addiction, the more impaired the patient's functioning in areas of work or school, relationships, finances, and job performance. The CAP asks whether the patient has missed days of work or school due to cocaine use; lost productivity in work or school; been fired or expelled; gotten into debt; exhausted savings; been arrested; been involved in any cocaine-related car accidents; stolen from work, family or friends, or elsewhere; become violent; had an important relationship break up due to cocaine; or become socially isolated.

Effects on sexual functioning should also be explored. Cocaine is often taken initially for aphrodisiac effects and its ability to enhance sexual functioning. As the chronic user becomes tolerant to these effects, he/she eventually finds that cocaine impairs rather than improves sexual performance. Some treatment applicants report that they have used cocaine as a "cure" for low sexual desire, impotence or frigidity, or to increase sexual endurance, prolong erections, and reduce inhibitions. But all of these effects are short-lived. Chronic users more often report impotence, failure to achieve orgasm, and a complete loss of sexual desire, and say that using cocaine has become an inhibitor rather than facilitator of sexual activity.

PSYCHIATRIC ILLNESS

Among cocaine addicts who present for treatment, a significant number exhibit symptoms of psychiatric illness, but most of these are temporary and secondary to the drug use itself. Because of its disruptive effects on the user's brain function and behavior, chronic cocaine use can make it very difficult to conduct an accurate psychiatric assessment of the patient. It is best to wait until he/she has been abstinent from all drugs for a period of several days or weeks. The effects of the cocaine crash and of long-term dopamine depletion resulting from chronic cocaine use can generate behavior and affective states that mimic a wide range of psychiatric illnesses, including depression, bipolar disorders, and anxiety disorders. Symptoms can include dysphoria, anergia, anxiety, sleep and appetite disturbances, and sexual disinterest. These cocaine-induced depressive symptoms often disappear without intervention within a week or two of stopping cocaine use.

Also common among chronic high-dose users is a short-term cocaine-induced psychotic state virtually indistinguishable from paranoid psychoses unrelated to drug use. Symptoms may include paranoid delusions, auditory or visual hallucinations, dysphoria, agitation and confusion, deterioration of personal hygiene, and sometimes suicidal or violent behavior. Acute symptoms of cocaine-induced psychosis tend to be transient and usually disappear within two to five days after the drug us stops. However, sometimes chronic high-dose cocaine use precipitates an underlying and possibly preexisting but formerly unexpressed psychosis that persists even in the absence of any drug use.

All treatment applicants should be asked to give a detailed account of the specific negative effects cocaine use has had on his/her mood or mental state, such as irritability, short temper, depression, memory problems, heightened suspicion of others, anxiety, panic attacks, paranoid thoughts, visual or auditory hallucinations, suicidal or violent impulses. Has the patient ever been hospitalized for psychiatric treatment, and if so for what types of problems? Has the patient ever consulted a psychiatrist, psychologist, or other mental health professional, and if so for what reason and with what results?

The prescription of psychotropic medications during the initial assessment is generally contraindicated for most presenting psychiatric symptoms for two reasons: First, drug-induced psychiatric effects are typically not very responsive to psychotropic medications. Second, premature introduction of medication can severely handicap the accuracy of psychiatric assessment and diagnosis. Patients who pose serious clinical management problems because they are psychotic, suicidal, or otherwise dangerous to themselves or to others need to be hospitalized immediately, and there, if indicated, appropriate psychotropic medication can be given without hesitation. In general, cocaine addicts who are suitable for outpatient treatment will not have psychiatric symptoms severe enough to warrant immediate use of psychotropic medication.

Excluding the transient cocaine-induced symptoms described earlier, the incidence of severe psychiatric disorders among cocaine addicts tends to be low. Among the minority of cocaine addicts who do have a history of psychiatric illness, the most common preexisting problems include depressive disorders, bipolar disorders, anxiety disorders, and severe narcissistic and/or borderline personality disorders.

Other Assessment Issues

SUPPORT SYSTEMS

Identifying the patient's existing or potential social support system helps to pinpoint available resources or, in some cases, areas of potential difficulty. Does the patient have the support of significant others, such as a spouse, other family members, or friends? Does the patient have a social network of friends who do not use drugs? Does the patient come in frequent contact with others who use drugs (through work, drug-dealing, and so on)? Does the patient have alternative sources of gratification with which to fill the gaps created by stopping cocaine use, such as an interest in sports or hobbies? Is the patient willing to attend self-help group meetings where he will find a ready-made support system, or is this unlikely? Identifying and mobilizing the patient's support system are crucial as part of early treatment efforts.

STRENGTH OF DRUG URGES AND CRAVINGS

The applicant's severity of cocaine addiction is closely related to the strength and frequency of cocaine cravings experienced between instances of cocaine use. Questions aimed at assessing this include the following: Do you have trouble turning down cocaine whenever it is offered to you? Does the sight, thought or mention of cocaine trigger urges and cravings for the drug? Are you often preoccupied with thoughts about it? Does the mere thought of cocaine almost always lead you to buy it and use it? Is there anything that stops you from using it when you get an urge or craving?

Urine Testing in Assessment

A urine sample obtained in the first visit verifies which drugs the applicant has used within the preceding several days. Test results may confirm the patient's verbal report of recent drug use or identify additional unreported drug use. A urine test can only identify the presence of drugs used within the most recent few days and tells nothing about the extent or frequency of use. Because cocaine is such a short-acting drug, its metabolites can be detected in the urine for only two or three days after last use in most instances. By contrast, the metabolites of marijuana can be detected for a much longer time after last use, sometimes for as long as 30–40 days in a chronic daily or almost daily user. Even occasional marijuana use can yield a positive test result for a week or longer.

TREATMENT CONTRACTING

Rationale and Benefits

The initial assessment interview should culminate in the formulation and signing of a written treatment contract which outlines the basic treatment plan and requirements of the program. A properly designed treatment contract can be an extremely valuable treatment tool.

The treatment contract should not be used merely to extract total compliance from a patient in a controlling or punitive manner. Unfortunately, many people have come to think of treatment contracting as a way of forcing addicts to maintain abstinence by getting them to agree to the imposition of harsh, irreversible, or even life damaging consequences if and when they fail to live up to the letter of the contract. Such contracts are not only ineffective, but also place the clinician in the impossible bind of trying to be both helper and executioner.

If outside persons or agencies choose to impose consequences on the addict who relapses or prematurely drops out of treatment, so be it; such limits are often necessary for the protection of others. But the clinician or program should not be involved in this process. For instance, in cases where a positive urine test is slated to result in job termination, suspension of a license, or other adverse consequences to the patient, the urine test should be taken by the outside agency, not by the treatment program. Urine tests taken by the program must be used for clinical purposes and clinical purposes only! To help, not hurt, must be the single focus of the clinician and the program.

The treatment contract should never be used to bludgeon the patient or to justify punishment for noncompliance, but rather to serve as a clear statement of treatment goals and expectations and to provide realistic feedback regarding any discrepancy between stated intentions and actions. Unkept treatment contracts highlight areas of denial and self-sabotaging "setups." For example, when the patient in early recovery reports involvement with certain friends identified as "high risk" in the treatment contract, the clinician can refer to the contract to point out the discrepancy in a way that helps the patient see his/her own reemerging denial more clearly.

The very process of establishing the contract serves a vital function. The way a patient responds to the treatment contracting process itself is often diagnostic and prognostic about his/her readiness for treatment. A treatment applicant who emphatically states a desire to stop using cocaine but bargains, for example, to have a treatment contract with few counseling sessions, no urine testing, and exemption from other program requirements, can be helped to see this clear-but behavioral evidence of his/her resistance and denial. Another applicant may agree without hesitation to every detail of the contract and express nothing but fierce motivation to comply with every aspect of the program but act out unexpressed ambivalence by demonstrating very little behavioral follow-through. Again, the written treatment contract validates the inconsistency and enables the clinician to address the denial, the ambivalence, and the self-destructive behaviors. This may lead the patient closer to self-awareness and willingness to cooperate more fully in his/her own treatment. The point here is that the treatment contracting process clarifies the requirements, realities, and rigors of treatment so that these issues can be squarely faced. The patient is better informed about what treatment involves and can make a more informed choice about whether to accept or decline the challenge.

Content of the Contract

Some of the basic items in the treatment contract include the following:

(1) The stated frequency of individual, group, and family counseling sessions.
(2) The stated time commitment to complete the program and a stipulation that any intentions by the patient to drop out of treatment prematurely will be aired for discussion before he/she follows through on this intention.
(3) A list of family members and significant others who can be alerted if the patient relapses, fails to show up for appointments, or drops out of treatment prematurely.
(4) The stated frequency of supervised urine testing performed each week and the requirement to give an additional urine sample whenever requested.
(5) An agreement to respect the confidentiality of all other patients in the program and to not divulge the identity of other patients to anyone outside the program.
(6) The stated frequency of self-help meetings that the patient must attend every week.
(7) An agreement to become totally abstinent from all drugs, including alcohol and marijuana, even if the patient doesn't feel that this is necessary for his/her recovery.

(8) An agreement to make telephone contact with at least one other member of the program every week.

(9) The identification of high-risk people, places, and things to be avoided during early recovery.

(10) An agreement to have family members or significant others be involved in the treatment program.

(11) An agreement to accept a referral to residential treatment facility if he/she is unable to achieve initial abstinence, comply with the basic requirements of the outpatient program, and/or show evidence of sufficient treatment progress.

The above items are suggested guidelines for possible inclusion in the treatment contract and do not represent an exhaustive list. No single treatment plan will be appropriate for all treatment applicants. In recent years, as cocaine use has spread to virtually all segments of the population, addicts seeking treatment have become an increasingly heterogeneous subgroup. While the same basic elements of effective treatment are often applicable to many different types of patients, certain aspects must be individualized to meet each patient's specific needs.

Introducing the Requirement of Total Abstinence

To the surprise of many clinicians, most patients feel greatly relieved to learn that there will be clearly enforced limits and accountability supported by urine testing, but more often they are highly resistant to giving up their "soft" drugs - alcohol and marijuana. Education about the nature of addictive disease may help the patient see the need for total abstinence, but rarely is this concept embraced wholeheartedly at the very outset of treatment. Sometimes it helps to ask the patient to proceed with total abstinence at least temporarily on "blind faith" until he/she has a better opportunity to see the benefits of this approach.

Patients should leave the first interview with the following behavioral assignments to help them establish initial abstinence:

(1) Discard all drug supplies and paraphernalia immediately upon returning home; if possible do this with the assistance of a family member or friend in order to block the temptation to get high again just "one last time."

(2) Immediately sever relationships with all drug dealers and users.

(3) Return to the program tomorrow.

Defining Clinician and Patient Roles

Patients must be helped to give up their wish to be "cured" by the therapist or program. The clinician's role is not to stop the patient from using drugs or take over responsibility for any continuation of the problem. The clinician cannot stand in the way of drug dealers or be available every time drug urges and cravings occur. The clinician *can* provide some of the tools that have been found to reliably help others become abstinent and recover, but it is up to the patient to make use of them.

The relative roles of the clinician and patient in the recovery process can be likened to that of a guide and a climber on a hiking trail. The role of the guide is just that — to guide, not carry the climber along the trail, to keep the climber safely moving in the right direction, to keep him/her on the right trail, to point out the dangers and pitfalls along the way, and to provide some of the basic tools or equipment needed to complete the climb. But the climber him/herself will have to take each and every step on the climb and exert his/her own energy and determination in order to reach the desired destination.

It is recommended that the treatment contract include the following statement: "I agree that I must take responsibility for my own recovery. I can use my counselor and program as tools to help me remain abstinent, but any return to drug use is my own personal choice and responsibility — and mine alone. No one can make me recover and no one can make me get high, if I don't want to."

Chances for Success

Which cocaine addicts are most likely to succeed in outpatient treatment? This is not an easy question to answer. Even the most experienced clinician has no crystal ball for making reliable predictions; however, my own clinical findings suggest a number of factors that are associated with better treatment outcomes. These include:

(1) Cocaine addicts who seek treatment voluntarily, with open recognition of the problem, its consequences, and its severity, do better than those who come to treatment under severe external pressure or coercion from family, court, or employer, and deny or minimize the extent of their drug problem and its consequences.

(2) Cocaine addicts who take personal responsibility for their recovery do better than those who place the responsibility on the program or clinician to supply a "quick-fix" cure.

(3) Cocaine addicts who have a history of good functioning, including stable employment, stable home life, and the absence of serious psychiatric problems before getting addicted to cocaine, do better than those who have a history of erratic functioning, crisis-ridden lives, tumultuous and destructive relationships, and use of many different drugs to self-medicate extreme chronic depression, dysphoria, or other negative mood states.

(4) Cocaine addicts who demonstrate a willingness and an ability to comply behaviorally with the basic program requirements during the first few weeks, especially with regard to punctuality, attendance, and follow-through on advice and suggestions from professionals and peers, do better than those who bargain for streamlined treatment plans and insist on doing almost everything their own way.

CHAPTER 7

Achieving Abstinence

COMPLETELY STOPPING THE USE OF cocaine and all other mood-altering substances is the first and foremost goal of outpatient treatment. Neither the addiction problem itself nor related problems and crises can be dealt with effectively until a period of abstinence is achieved.

The techniques for stopping compulsive cocaine use are similar to those used in eliminating other types of habitual and compulsive behaviors. The first task is to identify and break the chain of specific behaviors, thoughts, moods, feelings, etc., that perpetuate the vicious cycle of compulsive drug use. Insight-oriented techniques which attempt to uncover the psychological reasons why the addict is still using cocaine (or began using it in the first place) are not only ineffective but actually sabotage efforts to achieve abstinence by stirring up strong negative feelings that send the addict right back to drugs.

The following are essential steps to successfully achieving abstinence:

(1) Identify external cues and internal feeling states that trigger drug cravings and plan ways to avoid them.

(2) Establish a support system, daily structure, and substitute rituals to break the compulsive cycle of drug use and drug-related activities.

(3) Develop specific action plans for handling cravings and urges.

(4) Provide education about the role of conditioning factors in compulsive drug use.

(5) Formulate specific strategies to prevent premature dropout.

IDENTIFYING COCAINE CUES

As a result of having used cocaine literally hundreds or thousands of times in many different settings and circumstances, the addict's daily life becomes filled with numerous reminders of cues that trigger drug cravings and drug use. Most of these cues involve people, places, things, and emotional states associated with getting and using cocaine.

The strongest cue is likely to be the sight of cocaine itself. It is essential to ask patients whether they have any remaining or "forgotten" supplies of cocaine or hidden "stashes" in their home, car, office, etc., and to predict how and where they would be most likely to encounter cocaine "accidentally." They should be asked, "Even if you don't actively try to find cocaine, how is it likely to find you? Will your dealers call you if they don't hear from you? Which individuals whom might you run into in the next few days would offer you drugs?" In addition to dealers, anyone with whom the patient often used cocaine represents a potentially powerful cue. This may include friends, lovers, acquaintances, coworkers, family members, employers, and others. Just seeing pictures of cocaine or people using it in magazines, newspapers, movies, or television can provoke strong desires to get high.

Having a lot of cash, a credit card, or a checkbook can set off intense cravings for cocaine. One patient in his second week of abstinence revealed that he had been keeping a thousand dollars in cash in his pants pocket every day to test whether he was really committed enough to resist the intensely powerful drug urges that were set off every time he touched the wad of bills. Although he successfully resisted these urges at least several times, he finally gave in and used cocaine the day before recounting this setup for self-sabotage.

Drug paraphernalia that is part of the addict's cocaine use ritual can elicit drug cravings just as powerful as those elicited by the sight of cocaine itself. Paraphernalia may include freebase pipes, butane torches, coke spoons, coke inhalers or "bullets," coke vials and other miniature storage vessels, brass and gold-plated coke straws and razor blades, mirrors and marble slabs (for laying out "lines" of cocaine powder), "stash" boxes (for hiding drug supplies), and syringes or "works." There is also the equipment used to prepare "homemade" freebase such as baby bottles, pyrex glassware, and baking soda, ammonia, or ether.

Certain places where the patient frequently used cocaine, such as discos, bars, afterhours clubs, brothels, and hotels, become strong reminders of the drug. Some patients have habitually used cocaine at the office, in the office bathroom or lounge, in their car, or in a particular room in their own home. One patient, for example, typically used cocaine either in the back storeroom of his retail store or in the basement of his home. These two places provided him with plenty of secret hiding spots for cocaine and the privacy to use it any time of the day or night—shielded from the suspicious and watchful eyes of his wife.

A particular part of town, a particular street, or a particular building associated with places where the addict purchased and/or used cocaine can set off powerful urges and cravings for the drug. The mere sight of a highway exit sign can send the addict's car on "automatic pilot" right to the dealer's house, as described by a patient who fell victim to this reaction:

Every time I went on the highway between my home and office, I had to pass the exit to the dealer's house. During the first two weeks of the program, I found myself getting off at that exit every evening after work, without even realizing it. I would be in a trance and then wake up at the end of the exit ramp or sometimes not until I was already driving down his street. The pull was extremely powerful—I felt like a preprogrammed robot. The first couple of times I caught myself and drove away. Eventually I gave in. Before I knew what happened, I was sitting in his living room snorting lines and leaving with a little 'package' to get me through the rest of the night. It was scary.

Certain feeling states can be powerful cues for cocaine use. Boredom can be especially dangerous. During periods of free time, in the absence of planned activities, the addict's mind is likely to wander toward thoughts of cocaine: "If I just had some cocaine, just a little bit, I'd be having a good time." Other triggers for cocaine may include performance anxiety in a social or work situation; feeling depressed, lonely, angry, irritable, or frustrated; feeling happy, joyous, sexually aroused, or in a "party" mood. The desire for cocaine can be triggered just as easily (if not more so) by positive as well as negative moods. Feeling sexually aroused is often a strong drug cue for those who have used the cocaine to enhance normal sexuality, self-medicate preexisting sexual dysfunction/compulsions, or overcome sexual anxiety. For example, one patient reported that whenever he was with a new girlfriend with whom he anticipated having sex he would experience strong fantasies and urges for cocaine because he had for ten years always relied on the drug in this situation. Meeting new girlfriends was for him a highly predictable and powerful trigger for cocaine.

Cocaine cues can also include certain memories, anniversaries, holidays, sensations and experiences. For example, while in a laundromat, one patient was overwhelmed by cravings for cocaine in response to the smell of ammonia (a chemical he had used in preparing homemade freebase). Another patient experienced cravings whenever he heard songs on the radio performed by a particular rock group whose music he often listened to while high on cocaine. A birthday, a significant anniversary (such as the death of a loved one), a holiday associated with "partying" (such as Christmas, New Year's, July 4th, St. Patrick's Day), or a celebration (such as wedding, office party, job promotion) can all set off overwhelming desires for cocaine.

It is impossible to predict all of the addict's current or anticipated cocaine cues. The link between the subtlest cues and the urge to use cocaine can be deep, powerful, and outside of conscious awareness. While some cues appear without warning or anticipation, most can be identified. This is essential to the task of successfully breaking the cycle of compulsive drug use.

Keeping a running log or diary of cocaine-related thoughts and cravings is a good way for patients to heighten their awareness of personal drug cues. Patients are encouraged to write down specific circumstances immediately preceding the onset of cravings — how intense they are, how long they last, what thoughts or actions they stimulate about obtaining or using drugs, and what strategies are used to deal with them.

AVOIDANCE STRATEGIES

It is not enough merely to identify cocaine cues and triggers. Nor is it at all advisable for the patient to note cues and then purposefully expose him/herself to them in order to "build up resistance or test control" (like the patient who kept a wad of bills in his pocket). This battle of willpower is inevitably a losing one for anyone addicted to cocaine. The struggle is difficult enough without adding self-imposed handicaps.

The active cocaine addict who wants to stop using cocaine must do everything and anything possible (within reason) to avoid cocaine cues, reminders, and sources of access to the drug.

Discarding All Drug Supplies and Paraphernalia

If the patient has not already done this prior to the first interview, then specific plans immediately to get rid of all drugs (including marijuana, alcohol, pills, etc.) and all drug-related paraphernalia and other materials must be discussed and finalized before the end of the interview. These items should not be sold or given to friends, but destroyed and/or discarded in a way that immediately relieves the addict of having them in his/her possession and makes them permanently inaccessible. Drugs can be flushed down the toilet. Paraphernalia can be smashed and thrown in the garbage, preferably out of the addict's sight and reach. It is strongly advised that a non-drug-using friend or family member assist in this "search and destroy" mission in order to thwart any temptation by the addict to use "just one last time." For some patients, this task is simply too dangerous; they should let someone else do it for them. In the words of one such patient:

> I just couldn't deal with the thought of once again seeing cocaine, my freebase pipes, my kitchen cabinets stocked with baking soda. I knew it would set me off. There would be no stopping me. So instead I sent my father on a mission to get rid of everything while I waited outside in the car. Just knowing what he was doing gave me urges, but I was able to control it as long as I didn't have to stare all of those things right in the face.

Patients must be advised to discard all, not just some, of their paraphernalia. Many secretly hold onto certain cherished items in their collection:
"At first I didn't throw out every bit of my paraphernalia. I kept a little memento — a collector's item — just to remind me of my foolishness, so I thought. When I finally admitted this to my counselor, he said I was playing with fire — trying to keep my relationship with cocaine alive and to keep the door open for an easy return to the drugs and sex scene. I guess he was right. I went back and threw out the little rubber fixture from my freebase pipe, a porno tape that would set off my sexual compulsion, and the phone numbers of prostitutes and dealers. I felt much relieved having one more set of temptations gone."

Breaking Contact With Dealers and Users

It is impossible for patients to successfully stop using cocaine while they continue to maintain connections with dealers and users. The temptations will simply be too great. Although some newly abstinent patients proudly proclaim having refused cocaine in the presence of others who were using the drug and interpret this as an indication of their strong determination to stay clean, repeated exposure to these temptations erodes their determination and ultimately leads to their surrender.

Breaking off with dealers and users can be especially difficult when patients regard these people as valued "friends" even though the relationships revolve entirely around drugs. This dilemma is exemplified in the following statement made by a patient several months after stopping cocaine:

The person I had the most trouble breaking off with was a guy I considered my best friend in life. My counselor warned me, but I just didn't listen until I saw the problem for myself. I thought that I could still hang out with him and not get high. I figured that he would look out for my best interest and not let me get high with him. I was wrong. To make a long story short, I didn't get high the first couple of times I saw him after starting the program, but after watching him get high in front of me four or five times, I pleaded with him to let me have some — and he did. The next day, while talking about it with my counselor, I finally realized that my 'good buddy' wasn't really much of a friend at all. Anyone who uses cocaine in front of you when they know you have a problem and that you want to stop using is not your friend. He cared more about cocaine than he did about me. It hurt to face that fact and accept it, because he'd been my closest friend since high school. I thought we were like brothers, but we had become nothing more than drug buddies. When we weren't getting high we really didn't have much to say to each other. It's a sad realization — hard cold fact that I just had to face in order to get straight.

Other tough decisions arise when users and dealers include a mate, a sexual partner, a coworker, or a family member. Some patients have to change jobs, temporarily separate from a spouse or lover, or permanently end relationships with people who refuse to stop using cocaine. Significant others who are themselves involved with cocaine should be encouraged to seek help or otherwise stop their drug use as a precondition for continuing their relationship with the patient who has entered treatment.

Avoiding "High-Risk" Places

A patient reported that he lived just around the corner from the disco where he had become addicted to cocaine. For the preceding three years, he had spent four or five nights every week getting high there. During his first week of being abstinent from cocaine he noticed that every time he passed by the club on the way home, the mere sight of the club's door and the marquee set off powerful cravings and urges for cocaine. He considered moving to avoid this problem, but said he simply couldn't afford it. With the help of his counselor, he came up with a plan to reliably avoid the sight of the disco by taking a different route home — to approach his apartment building from the opposite direction even though it meant having to go several blocks out of his way. He felt that the added inconvenience was a small price to pay for avoiding the powerful cocaine cues.

Saying "No" Effectively

Many patients feel "put on the spot" when faced with an offer of drugs or alcohol that is either unexpected or made in the company of people with whom the addict feels self-conscious about not using. Developing effective ways to say "no" in advance of such offers can help. (After refusing the offer, the patient should immediately leave the situation, if at all possible.) Patients are asked to prepare at least two or three face-saving but definite ways to decline offers of alcohol and drugs. For example: "No thanks, I get a bad reaction to that." "No thanks, I don't do that anymore." "No thanks, I have a problem with that." "No thanks, I'm sorry but I have to leave now."

ESTABLISHING STRUCTURE, SUPPORT, AND ACCOUNTABILITY

The patient's desire to stop using cocaine must be translated into a specific plan of behavioral action. Giving up a drug-centered life is not just a mental exercise but an operational, behavioral task. A basic structure and daily routine (substitute ritual) must be offered to immediately replace the lifestyle dominated by seeking, using, and recuperating from cocaine. Structure, stability, and predictability are provided by a simple plan that patients can follow on a day-to-day basis—a framework and set of instructions for achieving abstinence. Healthy rituals and positive habits must replace destructive ones.

The clinician must be both directive and supportive in educating, encouraging, instructing, and advising the patient. In short, the clinician should be the armchair coach of the patient's daily activities. A firm but gentle and accepting "take charge" posture is called for here. Neither a passive analytic stance nor a harsh, judgmental, or overly controlling one will work effectively.

The basic structure for achieving abstinence includes the following:

(1) A SHORT-TERM GOAL

In most cases, a first full week of complete abstinence from all drugs is set as an immediate and reasonably achievable goal. For binge users, the comparable goal is to achieve a period of abstinence approximately twice as long as the usual time period between successive binges. This is defined as the first hurdle. For example, if binges are typically separated by two weeks, then the immediate goal is four weeks of total abstinence. The patient will probably experience increased cravings and urges at the two-week point and require extra structure and support to avoid cocaine use and resumption of the usual binge cycle. Setting realistic, short-term goals helps patients to stay focused on accomplishments within reach rather than on the seemingly impossible and overwhelming task of never using drugs again. Patients who succeed in achieving their first abstinence goal benefit form an early sense of reward and accomplishment. This builds positive momentum, bolsters feelings of self-control, counteracts defeatist attitudes, and reinforces other positive actions.

(2) FREQUENT COUNSELING SESSIONS

For at least the first week or two of treatment, the patient is seen as frequently as possible, usually daily or almost daily for brief (30-minute) individual counseling sessions to provide accountability, support, and encouragement. These sessions play a key role in structuring the patient's time, reinforcing the goal of immediate abstinence, and establishing a solid working alliance between patient and clinician. The events of the preceding 24 hours are reviewed in each session and advice or suggestions are given for safely getting through the next 24 hours.

(3) FREQUENT URINE TESTING

A supervised urine sample is taken every two or three days to verify abstinence or detect any unreported drug use. Urine testing establishes behavioral accountability for drug use and is seen by most patients as a backstop and an objective indicator of progress.

(4) OTHER EXTERNAL CONTROLS

While no one can control the addict and stop him/her from using drugs if he/she really wants to, there are a number of external controls in addition to urine testing that can be extremely useful in blocking the possibility of an impulsive return to drug use. These include placing patients' financial affairs (including bank accounts, credit cards, etc.) temporarily in the hands of responsible family members or friends; establishing curfews and procedures for check-in calls; obtaining a prior written commitment from patients to accept a referral to inpatient treatment should they relapse chronically and/or prematurely terminate outpatient treatment. Often patients' desire to avoid hospitalization and the resulting disruption and embarrassment increases motivation to achieve abstinence on an outpatient basis.

(5) A SOLID SUPPORT SYSTEM

It's not easy to stop using drugs alone. Establishing and utilizing a solid support system are just as important as avoiding drugs and drug cues. After completing their first two or three days of abstinence, new patients in our intensive outpatient program enter a beginner's recovery group. The group provides a ready-made support network and a forum for discussing early abstinence problems (e.g., drug cravings, environmental triggers) and how to deal with them (e.g., avoidance and coping strategies). Additional support, encouragement, and structure are provided by attending CA, AA, or NA meetings on a daily or almost daily basis (attending 90 meetings in 90 days is strongly recommended to new members). The patient is encouraged to identify and link up with a social network of non-drug-using friends, perhaps to rekindle those healthy social and family ties that suffered as a result of the active addiction. The support system also includes a special "buddy" (whether a family member, friend, or sponsor in a self-help group) to call in times of crisis or need.

(6) TIME PLANNING

It is potentially dangerous for the newly abstinent patient to spend much free time alone or to have large blocks of time during the day or evening without planned activities. Keeping busy reduces opportunities for using or fantasizing about drugs and avoids the common tendency to gravitate (often unconsciously) toward high-risk situations. Each day must be carefully scheduled and planned, in advance, in a log or appointment book that is reviewed with the clinician at every visit. The patient is encouraged to plan time for recreational activities, physical exercise, and social activities with "safe" people who are part of the patient's identified support system. This is especially important before weekends, holidays, and whenever one or more days are expected to lapse between counseling sessions.

HANDLING CRAVINGS AND URGES

Drug hunger — the impulsive and frequently overwhelming cravings and urges for cocaine — can and do occur despite perfect compliance with treatment plans and a sincere desire to remain drug free. Strong cravings can be especially difficult for patients to deal with when they are unprepared or the feelings occur unexpectedly, without warning. Patients are educated about how conditioning factors can elicit drug hunger and are taught how they can deal with the cravings and urges that are as a natural part of early abstinence. Patients are provided with a basic understanding of conditioning phenomena and how these concepts can be specifically applied to their addiction to cocaine, as outlined in Table 7.1. Some strategies that patients can use to deal with a craving or urge for cocaine are listed in Table 7.2.

PREVENTING PREMATURE DROPOUT

Most patient dropouts occur during the first 30 days of treatment. Patients who remain in treatment and comply with the basic program requirements beyond this period significantly improve their chances of positive

TABLE 7.1
Conditioning Factors in Cocaine Use

1. Cocaine cravings are a predictable result of chronic cocaine use and usually continue long after the cocaine use is stopped.
2. Cocaine cravings can be triggered or set off by people, places, things, feelings, situations, etc., previously associated with cocaine use. Anything that is a reminder of cocaine can be a trigger for cocaine cravings.
3. Cocaine cravings tend to be strong during the early abstinence period and then fade away over time, but lose their power only when not reinforced by cocaine use. As abstinence progresses, cravings usually become less frequent and less severe.
4. The strength of cocaine cravings does not diminish merely through the passage of time, but rather as a person successfully and consistently refuses to give in to cravings each time they occur. Cravings lose their power little by little, each time the person does something other than take drugs in response to the craving—a process known as "extinction."
5. Complete abstinence from cocaine and all other drugs is the best way to insure the most rapid and complete extinction of cocaine cravings.
6. The extremely high potency of potential cocaine cravings in early abstinence means that it is extremely dangerous and inadvisable for the newly abstinent addict to purposefully expose him/herself to drug cues in an attempt to speed up the extinction process. The result is usually counter-productive and self-defeating: strong cravings are elicited, the patient is unable to resist them, he/she uses cocaine, and the cravings are strengthened by the drug use.
7. Determination and willpower are poor defenses against cravings—specific actions must be taken to counteract cravings and urges whenever they occur.
8. Cravings and urges are always temporary. They are usually fleeting sensations that last no more than a few minutes and tend to disappear quickly when immediate action is taken to remove oneself from the situation that has set off the craving response. It is wrong to think that once a craving begins its intensity will automatically increase to the point where using cocaine becomes unavoidable. Using cocaine at the peak intensity of a craving maximally reinforces the connection between cocaine and cravings and is the surest way to increase both the frequency and intensity of future cravings.

---

outcome. Preventing early dropout, therefore, is essential to treatment success.

Among the factors that contribute to prevent premature dropout are: (1) unrealistic expectations and lack of cocaine-specific education; (2) early "slips"; (3) a "cure me" attitude; and (4) unresolved personal crises.

Unrealistic Expectations

After a few days or more of abstinence and especially when no cravings or urges are present, many patients feel "cured" and no longer in need of treatment. Although some patients remain ridden with cravings and urges

TABLE 7.2
Methods for Handling Cocaine Cravings

1. Leave the situation you are in, if at all possible.
2. Get involved in an activity to deflect or "short-circuit" the urge—do physical exercise, take a walk, go to a movie, take a peaceful drive in the country.
3. Talk out the urge with someone who is understanding and supportive. Call or visit a friend, a fellow group member, your sponsor, your therapist, anyone who can help.
4. Go to a Cocaine Anonymous meeting.
5. Read recovery literature.
6. Read your list of reasons for wanting to quit cocaine.
7. Think about the negative effects of using cocaine.
8. Detach yourself from the urge. Pull back from the feeling and look at it as if you were an outside observer. Remember that the urge is a feeling, not an imperative to act out on the feeling. You do have a choice whether to use cocaine or do something to preserve your abstinence.

throughout the early abstinence period, others experience little or none of these problems until later in recovery. Cocaine is such a short-acting drug that patients often look and feel remarkably better and return to fairly normal functioning shortly after stopping cocaine use. It is very easy, therefore, for the patient to conclude either that the problem is resolved or that he/she has it sufficiently under control that continuing to invest time, money, or energy in a recovery program is no longer needed.

Cocaine-specific education is essential to counteracting unrealistic expectations and premature dropout during the early stage of treatment. Patients who are highly ambivalent about treatment are nonetheless often very curious about the medical and scientific aspects of cocaine use and will eagerly participate in discussions about the relevance of this information to their own experiences with the drug. During the 8-week intensive program, a rotating series of lectures, films, and educational handouts is combined with topic-oriented discussions on the physical and psychological effects of cocaine, as well as the individual and family dynamics of cocaine addiction, to provide useful information and at the same time to establish a working relationship with even the most resistant patient.

Although some patients are asymptomatic almost immediately after stopping cocaine use, others experience lingering aftereffects (cocaine "withdrawal"), such as insomnia, irritability, mood swings, emotional overreactivity (or instead, numbness), low energy, short attention span, anhedonia (inability to experience pleasure), lack of sexual desire, and extreme sensitivity to stress. A patient who experienced intense post-cocaine symptoms described her problems as follows:

My first thirty days were the worst. I was bouncing off the walls with crazy, shifting moods. One minute I felt fine and the next minute I was crying hysterically. A good deal of the time I was numb. I felt nothing or maybe just didn't know what I was feeling. I was in a haze. I got mad easily and flew off the handle. Everything annoyed me, even the smallest little problem. My boyfriend said that I was impossible to be with. Sex was the last thing on my mind. I got very scared for a while thinking that my condition was permanent. I couldn't imagine living such a depressing, unhappy existence. I said to myself: If this is what life is like without cocaine, no thanks. Eventually I came out of it—just as my counselor said I would. The thought that it was just temporary is what kept me going. Otherwise I probably would have given up and just gotten high again.

At the beginning of treatment, patients are educated about cocaine aftereffects and the fact that they are temporary. Since post-cocaine symptoms are due to the drug's disruptive neurochemical effects on brain functioning, any further use of cocaine will only perpetuate and intensify them. Physical exercise and proper nutrition appear to accelerate the disappearance of cocaine aftereffects. A daily regimen of certain vitamins (B and C, in particular) and amino acids (tyrosine, phenylalanine, and tryptophan) is recommended by some clinicians because these neurotransmitter precursors are thought to facilitate the replacement of dopamine, norepinephrine, and serotonin, which have been depleted during chronic cocaine use. However, no systematic studies have conclusively demonstrated the benefits of these "natural" remedies or of the pharmacologic agents such as tricyclic antidepressants, bromocriptine, or other medications being studied for their potential use in alleviating post-cocaine symptoms. Presently, education and supportive counseling coupled with physical exercise and planned leisure time activities offer the safest and most effective way to deal with this problem.

Early "Slips"

A "slip" must be addressed as an avoidable mistake, not as a tragic failure. Some patients are perfectionistic about their recovery. They feel totally defeated and humiliated by a single slip and, unless helped to place the slip in its proper perspective, are likely to drop out of treatment to avoid further embarrassment. Through a detailed (nonjudgmental) review of circumstances and feelings surrounding the slip, the clinician helps the patient identify exactly how it happened and what actions can be taken immediately to prevent it from happening again. Patients usually expect the clinician to be disappointed and rejecting in response to a slip. By maintaining a caring, empathic, but clear problem-solving posture the clinician can keep the patient focused on the task of avoiding further slips rather than fueling self-defeating feelings of guilt and frustration. Patients should be reminded that they, not the clinician, suffer as a result of their return to drug use.

How many slips are too many? It is not helpful to specify an exact number, but certainly when the pattern of cocaine use is not significantly reduced or eliminated within the first two or three weeks of treatment a change in treatment plan, including possible residential care, must be considered.

Sometimes early slips to cocaine are triggered by the use of alcohol or marijuana in those patients who have not yet accepted the need for total abstinence. This problem tends to be self-limiting. A slip to cocaine on the heels of alcohol or marijuana can be a "convincer" that removes the patient's resistance to total abstinence. Unfortunately lectures and warnings are sometimes not nearly as effective as an actual slip in overcoming resistance to total abstinence.

"Cure me" Attitude

Some patients leave treatment abruptly, frustrated by the fact that the program cannot spare them the sacrifice and effort required to achieve abstinence from cocaine. They have difficulty accepting personal responsibility for their own role in the treatment process and may become disappointed or angry when they experience an intense drug craving, use drugs, or encounter some other "rough spot" during early abstinence. They expect to be "fixed" by the program, as expressed in the following patient's statement:

> I went into treatment with the attitude of 'OK, I'm here, now fix me, cure me, do whatever you have to in order to get rid of this problem for me.' The way I saw it, if I just showed up for group and individual sessions, somehow the benefits of being there would just filter through to me and I'd be cured. I didn't do anything to change my lifestyle, the people I spent time with, or most of all my attitude. Soon enough my old drug buddies came over and before I knew it I was crashing from a two-day cocaine binge. When I came back to the program I was mad at everyone except myself: my counselor, the other group members, the doctor—why didn't they see what was going on and figure out a way to stop me? Wasn't that the purpose of the program—to stop me from getting high? What I got confronted with in group was my refusal to accept personal responsibility for using the tools offered by the program. I had plenty of options and I just didn't try to use any of them. I was just

sitting back and waiting to be fixed, like a car in for repairs. It was getting me nowhere. When I finally faced the problem squarely, accepted it, and made up my mind to do whatever I had to do in order to stay straight, everything went a lot smoother. It ended up being easier to place the responsibility on myself rather than continue to pass it off onto others. My change in attitude probably saved my life.

Unresolved Crises

Patients who continue to suffer marital, job, financial, or other personal crises during early abstinence often lose whatever motivation they may have had to give up cocaine in the first place. Even when the crisis has little or nothing to do with the patient's previous use of cocaine (which is rare), the resulting stress often stimulates intense cravings and supplies the patient with what he/she feels is a justification for continued drug use. Crisis intervention and supportive, directive counseling are often needed to clarify and resolve pressing problems. Even if the crisis cannot be resolved immediately, a clear statement of potential strategies for addressing the problem(s) can relieve a good deal of anxiety and thereby allow the patient to focus more intensively on achieving abstinence.

Sometimes family members are so angry, resentful, and mistrustful toward the newly abstinent patient that a crisis atmosphere is perpetuated at home. The patient may become discouraged with staying abstinent from cocaine when problems at home either stay the same or get worse in the absence of his/her drug use. Many say to themselves, "Why should I bother staying straight if my wife or my parent is still furious with me and accuses me of continuing to get high anyway?" Involving family members and significant others at the outset of treatment is often crucial in order to address immediate crises and stabilize the patient's home situation so that he/she can successfully stop using cocaine (see Chapter 10).

A WRITTEN PLAN FOR GETTING OFF COCAINE

Some of the basic suggestions and guidelines for achieving initial abstinence from cocaine are listed in Table 7.3. Each item asks the patient for a written response which is subsequently reviewed and discussed in group or individual sessions during the first few days of treatment.

As mentioned previously, the real goal of treatment is not just to get off, but to stay off cocaine—the focus of the next chapter, "Preventing Relapse."

TABLE 7.3
Guidelines for Getting Off Cocaine

1. Avoid all people, places and things associated with cocaine and other drugs. Write down the specific people, places, and things that could threaten your ability to stop using cocaine.
2. Choose a comfortable way to say "no" to offers and temptation to use cocaine. Write down three statements that you can use comfortably to refuse cocaine.
3. Identify your available support system—people you can spend "safe" time with and call in an emergency if you get an urge for cocaine. Write down the names and telephone numbers of at least five such people and keep the list with you at all times.
4. Spend as little free time as possible by yourself and without structured plans and activities to avoid trouble. Write down at least one "safe" activity for every evening or other period of free time this week. List substitute activities in case your original plans fall through.
5. Put all "heavy duty" personal problems on hold for right now. Your first priority is to stop using all drugs. Write down any personal problems that have been bothering you lately which should be addressed after you have stopped using cocaine.
6. Read at least 10 pages of recovery literature every day. Write down the names of at least one book/pamphlet you plan to read from every day this week.

CHAPTER 8

Preventing Relapse

ONCE PATIENTS HAVE achieved stable abstinence for at least several weeks, the focus of treatment shifts from getting off cocaine (and all other drugs) to staying off, that is, to preventing relapse. The 16-week relapse prevention phase of the intensive outpatient program is for patients who have completed either the initial eight-week intensive phase or a 30-day or longer residential treatment program.

The major goals of this phase are to prevent patients from having relapses, maintain abstinence, and lay the foundation for a lasting recovery. Education and counseling address attitudes and perceptions about relapse, early warning signs and relapse triggers, the need for improved coping skills to deal with addiction-related and other personal problems/stressors, and the need to move beyond an intellectual, verbal admission that the addiction problem exists to a deeper experiential acceptance of the problem and the need for personal change.

THE RELAPSE PROBLEM

When Mark Twain remarked, "It's easy to stop smoking—I've done it hundreds of times," he was referring, of course, to the problem of chronic relapse with regard to his own nicotine addiction—to the fact that stopping an addictive behavior is not nearly as difficult as staying off it permanently. Similarly, many cocaine addicts are able to stop using cocaine—for a few days, weeks, months, or even longer—but somehow end up using it again despite having made sincere and well-intentioned promises of permanent abstinence to themselves and others.

Relapse rates among cocaine addicts remain unnecessarily high, especially among those who leave residential care with a false sense of security (having been temporarily insulted from triggers and stressors) and without a highly structured relapse prevention program. Although relapse is the major stumbling block in addiction treatment, programs have traditionally avoided even mentioning it. Until recently, the occurrence of a relapse was actually considered treatment failure; understandably, perhaps, program staff who wanted to avoid communicating to patients potentially self-fulfilling expectations of failure saw relapse as a "dirty word." Treatment programs remained focused on detoxification and early abstinence issues and largely ignored the problem of preventing relapse and maintaining abstinence over the long term.

It is now openly accepted that relapses can and do happen, and that it is entirely possible for their occurrence to be minimized or even avoided completely. No one knows exactly what percentage of cocaine addicts successfully recover without any relapses whatsoever. Based on current knowledge, it is safe to assume that most patients relapse one or more times before achieving a state of stable, continuous abstinence. Some recovering addicts experience a single relapse (usually during their first year of abstinence), learn from it, redouble their efforts, and remain abstinent thereafter. Others experience a series of sporadic relapses interspersed between longer and longer periods of abstinence, with gradual improvement toward a more permanent drug-free state. Still others relapse repeatedly and continuously, after only brief periods of temporary abstinence, and never recover—or die. It is unlikely that relapse rates for treated cocaine addicts will ever be reduced to zero. Relapse continues to be a major contributor to unnecessary dropout, treatment failure, frustration of patients and their families, and staff burnout. Fortunately, however, specific relapse prevention strategies are helping to lower relapse rates significantly.

It is undoubtedly best to recover without any relapses. Short of that, the most desirable outcome is to have as few relapses as possible and as a result learn how to avoid them and how to recover most successfully thereafter. Recovering cocaine addicts should be helped to recognize the importance of continuous abstinence, but they should also be taught that a relapse is not the end of the world. It's an avoidable mistake. It's a signal that their efforts in recovery are incomplete and that some aspect of their plan to remain abstinent needs revision or supplementation.

MYTHS VS. FACTS ABOUT RELAPSE

Relapse is the process of returning to the use of cocaine or other drugs by a person who has remained abstinent for a period of time and has made a serious attempt at recovery. Patients who enter treatment for a short while, participate superficially, and then return to cocaine use have not relapsed — they have remained continuously addicted despite a fleeting period of abstinence. This underscores the fact that recovery requires personal changes that go far beyond just not using drugs; abstinence alone is not recovery. In order for a return to drug use to be considered a "relapse," the patient must have at least begun the recovery (change) process in the first place.

There are at least several damaging myths about relapse that are held by many patients and clinicians alike. Eliminating and correcting these myths are essential to utilizing relapse prevention techniques successfully. In fact, educating patients about the following myths and realities that surround the relapse phenomenon is itself an effective relapse prevention strategy.

Myth #1: Relapse Is a Sign of Poor Motivation

Although relapses can indeed be a sign of extreme ambivalence or poor motivation to give up cocaine, even the most highly motivated and sincere patients can have relapses. Change is risky. The outcome is often uncertain. It means giving up something that is known and familiar for something that may be unknown and unfamiliar. People in the process of changing their behavior are almost always ambivalent about giving up their old ways and adopting new ones. It can be very difficult to break habits, especially overlearned and multidetermined behaviors that are driven by a combination of biological, psychological, and social factors, as in the case of cocaine addiction. Moreover, the patient's ability to learn and successfully apply relapse prevention methods may sometimes lag behind the onset of powerful relapse cues that strongly challenge his/her ability to remain abstinent.

A lifelong (but reducible) vulnerability to relapse is considered to be a standard diagnostic feature of all addictions, and with cocaine addiction this vulnerability is especially strong. Relapse means that there is something wrong with the patient's recovery plan — not with the patient. A willingness to attempt the difficult task of personal change means a willingness to make mistakes and learn from them.

Myth#2: Relapse Is a Sign of Treatment Failure

Relapse is an avoidable mistake — a temporary interruption in the patient's abstinence — nothing more and nothing less. It has a beginning and an end. The assumption that having a relapse means that the patient is forever doomed to chronic, repeated drug use is false and damaging. Relapse means that the patient's recovery plan is incomplete. It is a signal that the patient is either doing something that he/she shouldn't be doing (such as overworking or spending time with old drug buddies) and/or not doing something that he/she should be doing (such as attending CA meetings or planning specific leisure time activities).

Although relapse must never be recommended to patients, it is essential that both clinicians and patients carefully examine any relapse episode for its potential learning value in preventing future relapses. But it is equally important to state explicitly that discussing relapse—accepting it as a possibility, preparing in advance to avoid a relapse, or examining its learning value—must not be construed by patients as permission to use drugs again or as an expectation that relapse is inevitable. By analogy, one can discuss the possibility of a medical emergency and learn in advance how to deal with it by practicing potentially life-saving first-aid techniques, without actually creating the emergency itself. Relapse is always potentially dangerous; when the addict returns to drugs and losses control, anything can happen, including serious injury or death.

Myth #3: Relapse Is Unpredictable and Unavoidable

Relapses do not just "come out of the blue." They never occur without prior warning, especially if the clinician, the patient, and significant others all know how to recognize early warning signs and take appropriate action. Because relapse is the endpoint of a stepwise progression of certain attitudes and behaviors that eventually lead back to drug use, there are always numerous opportunities to intervene. Relapses are avoidable.

**Myth #4: Relapse Occurs Only When Patients Use
Their Drug of Choice, in This Case, Cocaine**

Relapse means the use of any mood-altering addictive chemical, including alcohol and marijuana. A cocaine addict who fails to remain abstinent from these substances, even when this use is not compulsive or causing noticeable problems, is already well on the way toward relapse to cocaine. Refusing to accept the need for total abstinence is itself indicative of a relapse attitude.

**Myth #5: Relapse Is an Instantaneous Event That Occurs Only
When the Patient Actually Takes Drugs Again**

Returning to cocaine use is the endpoint, not the beginning, of the relapse process, as outlined below in the section on The Relapse Chain. Grasping this idea is central to successfully identifying early warning signs and devising strategies to prevent relapse.

Myth #6: Relapse Erases or Nullifies Whatever Positive Changes in Recovery Have Been Made Up To That Point

According to this myth, relapse either obliterates all progress or means that the progress was not really genuine in the first place—an idea with potentially devastating impact on the patient. Recovering addicts with many years of hard-earned, continuous abstinence can end up relapsing themselves into oblivion or death because they feel that all is lost. They experience intense guilt and shame and simply can't imagine starting all over again. In fact, to the extent that patients believe in this myth, the longer they have remained abstinent the more difficult it will be for them to overcome any relapse that might occur.

Relapse does not mean that the patient has lost everything and must start over again—especially if he/she continues in treatment rather than drops out, returns as quickly as possible to a drug-free state, and redoubles efforts to pick up the recovery process where he/she had left off and moves forward with even more determination than before. A temporary setback can provide invaluable information about the cause of the slip and ways to prevent it from recurring in the future.

Myth #7: The Absence of Relapse Guarantees Successful Recovery

Abstinence presents an opportunity to recover, but is not in itself a guarantee of recovery, nor does it mean that the addict is healthy and mature. The length of a patient's abstinence has little to do with the quality of his/her recovery. Some addicts never relapse but never make truly significant changes or achieve lasting growth or satisfaction in their lives; they remain stuck in repetitive, empty, or nonproductive lifestyles. Many others who do relapse make enormous strides in their personal growth and maturity and build reasonably happy, satisfying lives. Abstinence is a first step in recovery, but only a first step. By achieving stable abstinence, patients are freed from the preoccupation with drugs and can devote their time and energy to addressing the underlying disease of addiction—the deeply ingrained complex of maladaptive, self-defeating thoughts, attitudes, feelings, and behaviors that must be changed in order to successfully recover.

THE RELAPSE CHAIN: THE ROUTE BACK TO COCAINE

Relapse is a process, a progressive chain of behaviors, attitudes, and events that is initiated long before the patient actually starts using cocaine again. It's hard to pinpoint precisely where a relapse actually begins, but usually a major stressor or change (whether positive or negative) is the precipitant that sets the process in motion. The addict then fails to adequately address or cope with the stress; addictive thinking and behavior patterns are rekindled and/or intensified (including denial and social withdrawal); the problems and their resulting consequences or complications get worse; and the addict ends up feeling overwhelmed and "entitled" to use cocaine again.

The relapse chain can take many different forms, but might look something like this:

(1) A buildup or onset of stress caused by either negative or positive (but usually negative) changes and life events, (e.g., marriage, divorce, job change, job promotion, financial problems, financial gains).

(2) Activation of overly negative or positive thoughts, moods, and feelings, including confusion, bewilderment, irritability, depression, elation, or instead, complete numbness.

(3) Overreaction or total failure to take action in response to the situation or stress, leading to a perpetuation and escalation of problems.

(4) Denial that the problem is serious or even exists; failure to utilize one's existing support system and other tools of recovery. The patient fails to honestly share his/her feelings in counseling sessions or self-help meetings by remaining silent or presenting an incomplete or inaccurate picture to others. Attendance at meetings or counseling sessions becomes sporadic. Active drug cravings may or may not be experienced at this point.

(5) The original problems "snowball"—and new ones are created as the patient continues to categorically ignore them.

(6) The patient perceives the situation as being beyond the point of no return and feels totally incapable of doing anything about it. Positive thoughts about the "good times" on cocaine cross the patient's mind with increasing frequency. The idea of using cocaine looks increasingly appealing. Relapse seems entirely justifiable.

(7) The patient increasingly finds him/herself in high-risk situations or engaging in other subtle and not-so-subtle acts of self-sabotage. He/she has fleeing thoughts about obtaining and using cocaine, but still resists.

(8) Stress further increases as the patient's life continues to skid out of control while he/she becomes increasingly isolated and alienated from his/her support system. Frustration, despair, embarrassment, hopelessness, and self-pity set in and trigger obsessive thoughts about using cocaine.

(9) Irresistible cravings and urges lead the patient to obtain and use cocaine and/or other drugs. The relapse chain is complete.

RELAPSE RISK FACTORS AND WARNING SIGNS

Warning signs and risk factors always appear before the patient returns to cocaine or other drugs. The earlier these warnings are detected and brought to the patient's attention, the easier it is to take appropriate action and short-circuit the relapse chain before it culminates in drug use.

Relapse Attitudes and Thought Patterns

THE "PINK CLOUD" OR "HONEYMOON"

The dramatic, positive effects of stopping cocaine use can be striking — at least for a short while before the stress and problems of "real life" set in. When immersed in this "honeymoon," which typically occurs within the first two months of abstinence, patients tend to deny the existence of any life problems, negative feelings, or vulnerability to relapse; they find it difficult to believe that serious problems of any kind will resurface. Having given up cocaine, the true source of all their problems — so it seems — they can not live "happily ever after" by just continuing to remain drug free. Patients in this frame of mind are extraordinarily prone to overreacting to almost any problem that "bursts the bubble," no matter how large or small. They are at high risk for relapsing in response to overwhelming disappointment and surprise when unexpected problems arise.

NEGATIVE ATTITUDES: "STINKING THINKING"

There are certain negative attitudes and thought patterns that are classic, reliable signs of relapse. In the AA literature these attitudes are labeled "stinking thinking." In general, addictive or "stinking" thinking represents a reemergence or continuation of the addict's intense dependency needs, difficulty in facing problems, desire for immediate gratification, and tendency to focus on the negative. The addict continues to think, feel, and act addictively even though he/she is not using drugs — the so-called "dry drunk" pattern. A few "stinking" attitudes are described below.

(1) Still doubting that the addiction problem really exists: This attitude is often accompanied by various illusions: that the problem is limited to the use of only a single substance — cocaine; that the addiction was caused by problems no longer present; that determination and willpower alone will suffice in overcoming the addiction; and that life on cocaine never really became unmanageable in the first place. When the topic of relapse is discussed, the patient's response may include: "It won't happen to me," "I can control myself now," "I think I'm cured — the program has done wonders for me and you're the best therapist I've ever met," "Staying away from cocaine hasn't been nearly as difficult as I thought, I think I'm over this problem."

(2) Self-pity: "Why am I cursed with this problem?" "Why me?" "How

come others can get high, but I can't?" "It's just my luck, nothing ever goes right for me." When patients wallow in self-pity, continue to beat themselves up for being addicts, and remain unwilling to take definitive action to change, they inevitably keep themselves hovering on the brink of relapse.

(3) Impatience: "My recovery isn't going quickly enough." "Can't I graduate from this program sooner?" "Wouldn't it be better for me to just forget about my addiction and get on with my life?" "Only when I come to groups or go to CA meetings do I even think about cocaine—wouldn't I be better off just going to an exercise or meditation class instead of coming here to talk about my problems over and over again?" Patients who feel frustrated that their recovery is not proceeding at lightning speed are usually heading straight for relapse. "If life isn't getting better quickly enough without cocaine, why not go back to it?"

(4) Expecting too much from others: This is similar to the "cure me" attitude described in Chapter 6, where patients place the responsibility for their recovery on others and make unrealistic or even irrational demands on those around them. The patient is prone to feeling extremely angry, frustrated, and entirely justified in using cocaine when someone refuses to immediately and unequivocally grant a wish or satisfy a demand, no matter how unreasonable.

Patients in this frame of mind make the decision as to whether or not they will use drugs contingent upon the attitude and behavior of others. For example, some patients overreact when family members who have been victimized by the addiction remain suspicious and mistrustful. The patient often expects to be granted instant credibility and has difficulty accepting that he/she can earn back the family's trust only through consistent action. Often the patient's exaggerated expectations and resulting disappointment focus on the therapist and/or treatment program: "If the therapist was really doing his/her job, I wouldn't be having such a rough time," "Isn't this program supposed to help me recover with the least amount of pain and suffering?" It can be difficult for patients to confront their own personal responsibility for change and the fact that others cannot do it for them. It can also be difficult to confront long-standing or deep-seated dependencies, which challenge a facade of autonomy and independence. However, patients who fail to take responsibility for their recovery and place the burden too much on others remain precariously within arm's reach of relapse.

(5) Being negative, blaming, and chronically dissatisfied: Another feature of "stinking thinking" is being fiercely unhappy, negative, rejecting of all advice and attempts to console, and overly focused on other people's shortcomings, and blind to one's own problems and deficiencies. Often this is accompanied by a tendency to blame others and to feel that life is meaningless and empty. Patients who are operating in this self-defeating, "help-

rejecting complainer" mode are usually masterful at alienating people in their support system. Ultimately, this creates a seemingly perfect justification for relapse as they are left feeling overwhelmed, lonely, and "out on a limb," with no one around who cares.

(6) Overconfidence, grandiosity and defiance: Patients can feel overconfident to the point of actively putting themselves in dangerous, high-risk situations just to prove that they have become strong enough to resist temptation. Grandiosity and feelings of uniqueness as part of a relapse pattern lead patients to behave as it the ordinary laws that govern the universe do not apply to them—others may need to attend self-help meetings, therapy sessions, and give supervised urines, but not them. They are a special kind of addict—the kind that can recover without admitting vulnerability, adhering to total abstinence, or accepting help from others. Defiance is a natural outgrowth of these attitudes. The patient may appear perfectly pleasant, agreeable, and at least pseudo-complaint, but remains resentful, rebellious, and highly skeptical. Inevitably, the defiance becomes more obvious as the discrepancy widens between what the patient is advised to do and promises to do on the one hand, and what he/she actually does on the other.

(7) Life can't be fun without drugs: Patients who fail to make positive changes in their lifestyle or to fill the void left by cocaine with healthy, pleasurable activities are likely to confirm their own expectations that life is boring and meaningless without drugs. While actively addicted to cocaine, many patients totally avoid leisure time activities; others engage in certain activities, but only while under the influence of cocaine. Learning how to have a good time without drugs can be an anxiety-provoking experience. Also, so-called "natural highs" are not likely to duplicate the excitement, immediacy, and intensity of cocaine-induced highs.

(8) Rigid attitudes and beliefs: While providing seemingly simple solutions for complicated problems, rigid attitudes and belief systems interfere with the openness and flexibility required to build a meaningful life without drugs. Rigidly holding onto abstinence (called "white knuckling"), stubbornly refusing to accept advice, suggestions, or offers of assistance from others ("I'll do it my own way"), and refusing to let go of harmful, mistaken beliefs about addiction and recovery are all reliable signs of relapse. When patients are stuck in this mind set there is only one way to stay abstinent— their way. They are intolerant of differences of opinion and imperfection. They tend to be extremely harsh and judgmental toward peers who relapse, often unconsciously defending against their own impulses to get high again. When a patient who has held onto these rigid attitudes has a slip, he/she usually has an intense "boomerang" reaction, i.e., an extreme, self-incriminating defeatist reaction that leads to an extremely severe, dangerous relapse.

CHRONIC NEGATIVE MOODS AND FEELINGS

Chronic unresolved feelings of boredom, depression, loneliness, unhappiness, anger, anxiety, shame, and guilt, as well as painful and/or traumatic memories, are often precursors to relapse. Negative moods often follow the patient's realization that all of life's problems are not permanently resolved by stopping cocaine use. Eliminating drug and alcohol use leaves a large void or "gap" which can expose intense feelings of boredom and loneliness. Also, when cocaine is no longer present to chemically anesthetize and buffer other negative affects, such as anger and depression, patients often feel overwhelmed and experience the impulse to "self-medicate."

Many addicts have problems with anger and assertiveness. While chronically using cocaine, they become withdrawn and preoccupied and either avoid or ignore circumstances that would normally provoke anger. Those who were chronically anxious and unassertive before cocaine usually have severe difficulties responding appropriately in stressful interpersonal situations: They feel extremely angry at others for putting them in difficult situations and even angrier at themselves for not responding appropriately. Many act out these feelings in ways that backfire and make existing problems even worse — further increasing their self-justification for cocaine use.

Chronic depression can be a temporary aftereffect of chronic cocaine use, but it can also be a response to chronically unresolved situational or interpersonal stressors that must be addressed as part of the recovery plan. Some patients lose important relationships as a result of their addiction and experience extreme loneliness, guilt, and depression. Others return to jobs feeling stigmatized and ashamed because of previous drug-related behavior. Still others who are combat veterans or victims of disasters, rape, incest, parental addiction, near-fatal illness, or any type of trauma have difficulty living with painful memories and emotional scars that tend to surface abruptly and intensely, usually after a delay of several weeks or months after their drug use stops.

IDEALIZING THE COCAINE "HIGH"

Patients who continue to idealize or extol the pleasures of cocaine and selectively recall only good times on the drug are at increased risk for relapse. Known also as "euphoric recall," this phenomenon increases the patient's relapse potential by heightening the allure of cocaine and diminishing its perceived dangers — a reliable formula for feeding ambivalence about giving it up. "War stories," provocative, graphic accounts of "wild and wonderful" experiences on cocaine, provide a vivid example of selective memory and euphoric recall. Listening to these one-sided, romanticized versions of drug-induced highs can be a powerful relapse trigger, because it almost always stimulates intense cravings in other addicts who may be present as well as in the storyteller him/herself. "War stories" are dangerous and must be categorically avoided, especially in recovery groups. The tendency to selectively recall the good and forget the bad usually increases significantly when patients are feeling stressed or otherwise unhappy or uncomfortable, as evidenced in the following statement:

> I tend to idealize the cocaine high whenever I'm in a situation where I don't have control. When I just can't control something important in my life—a financial situation, a personal relationship, whatever—I think about the 'power' and control that I felt when doing cocaine, the power I thought I had. If I dwell on those good feelings too much, I get cravings. It's scary how easily I forget the horrors of cocaine—the eviction notices, the car accident, the overdue bills, the depression, the misery. Those negative thoughts go right out the window in a flash when I'm romanticizing the high.

DESIRE TO TEST CONTROL

Doing well in treatment for several weeks or months often stimulates fantasies about the possibility of returning to "controlled" cocaine use. When patients feel stronger, more in control of their lives, no longer victimized by bad moods, and free of the problems which led to their addiction, they often begin to rationalize that the time is right to try cocaine one more time, just to see if now they can control it. In the words of one patient:

> I thought I'd prove everyone wrong, so I went out and tested myself. I invented a little experiment to see if I could handle getting high again—in the back of my mind I figured that if I passed the first test, I could probably handle doing cocaine once in a while again. That would be a score—a real accomplishment. After all, I said to myself, my life was going fine, no big problems, no big worries, no cravings or urges to get high—the situation seemed perfect. Wrong! After the first test, I failed, I ended up on a four-day binge of cocaine and alcohol. Now I realize my 'test' was stupid. But it showed me that the addiction, the vulnerability, was still there even though my life seemed to be going fine.

This is, of course, an example of a self-sabotaging setup for relapse—one that patients often plan secretly unless the clinician is alert to this possibility and questions patients about it periodically.

DESIRE TO INDULGE

A patient's desire to indulge in cocaine again often comes on the heels of feeling deserving of a reward and relief for putting up with the stress and hassles of daily life or a particularly difficult problem. Some say retrospectively that they had intentionally let stress levels or problems build up to a point where using cocaine seemed entirely justified—"I deserve a break today."

POSITIVE MOODS

It is a grave mistake to focus only on negative feelings or events for signs of potential relapse. When feeling good, patients are prone to feeling a false sense of security about their addiction. They start believing that they can handle a drink, a toke, or a snort without getting out of control. They feel entitled to a reward.

RELATIONSHIP AND SEXUAL PROBLEMS

After several weeks or months of abstinence, patients may notice problems in their marriage or other intimate relationships that they had previously ignored, overlooked, or obliterated from consciousness with drugs. Moreover, family members who had become co-dependents locked into the "dance" of addiction may find it difficult to adjust to the now-abstinent cocaine addict and to the absence of a crisis-ridden lifestyle. They may become extremely angry, depressed, short-tempered, or otherwise difficult for the patient to get along with (see Chapter 10 for details). Paradoxically, peace and quiet at home can be threatening and anxiety-provoking. The children of patients in early abstinence often have a delayed reaction to the pain and suffering caused by their parents' previous drug use and irrational behavior.

Unresolved sexual problems can be extremely powerful relapse triggers. Many newly abstinent cocaine addicts experience a temporary loss of sexual desire, sometimes lasting for several weeks or months into early recovery. This apparent physiological aftereffect of chronic cocaine use can be misinterpreted by a mate as a sign of rejection or change of heart. Patients who have not had sober sex in many years may have intense fears and performance anxiety which can lead to temporary impotence, premature ejaculation, or failure to achieve orgasm. Many become terrified that the problem will become chronic or even permanent. Learning how to comfortably experience sexual feelings and intimacy without drugs can be a major accomplishment in preventing relapse to cocaine.

RELAPSE DREAMS

Drug dreams, especially recurrent and vivid ones, are usually very disturbing to patients in the first few weeks of recovery. Upon waking up from such dreams, patients often feel as though they have actually relapsed and may continue to feel guilty and disappointed in themselves for some time thereafter. Many patients tend to view drug dreams as prophetic—as indicating that they are not sufficiently motivated to stay drug free and are doomed to relapse: "If I have no intentions of getting high again, why would I do it in my dream?" Obviously, these feelings and unfounded beliefs can contribute to an actual relapse if allowed to fester. Since stress reactions do tend to stimulate drug dreams, exploring the circumstances surrounding the dream is valuable.

Relapse Behaviors

"BACK DOOR" SETUPS

Patients headed for relapse often put themselves in high-risk situations "accidentally" and encounter cocaine through the "back door." Through a series of subtle, self-sabotaging acts they create or find themselves in situations that virtually guarantee an encounter with cocaine, but in a way that appears to absolve them of any responsibility for having arranged the scenario. For example, the patient may accept a party invitation knowing full well that, although the host and hostess and most other invited guests do not use drugs (a seemingly "safe" and "respectable" gathering), at least one other person who is likely to attend will bring a supply of cocaine to share. In recounting the story later, the patient may emphasize what "bad luck" it was to run into a former cocaine-using friend who was sitting there getting high and how the temptation was "just too much to resist." "Back door" setups are indicative of the patient's continuing denial and difficulty in taking responsibility for protecting his/her own abstinence, as described by a female patient:

I used men as my setups, so I couldn't be blamed for a relapse. During my first few months in the program, I went out with guys who were actively using drugs. I'd go with them to cop, I'd watch them cook up the freebase, I'd sit and watch them get high. For a while, I refused over and over again to take even one hit on the pipe, just to prove that I was really trying to be 'good.' When I finally gave in, I deluded myself into thinking that it just wasn't my fault. It felt beyond my control, like I had nothing to do with setting it up—the guys I was spending time with were to blame—not me! So I thought. My denial was ten feet thick.

OVERREACTING TO SLIPS AND RELAPSES

The relapse myths and distortions mentioned earlier come to bear in an intensely negative way on patients who relapse after achieving a significant period of abstinence. What may have started as an isolated, contained "slip" escalates into a full-blown destructive relapse—a self-fulfilling result of the

patient's exaggerated negative reaction. This defeatist response is characterized by the following:

(1) Profound feelings of personal failure and the expectation of con-
    tinued failure.
(2) Feelings that all progress achieved before the renewed drug use is
    completely and forever lost.
(3) Feelings of self-hate and extraordinary disappointment for having
    submitted to temptation coupled with attribution of the drug use
    to personal weakness, lack of willpower, and low self-worth.
(4) Feelings of extreme ambivalence and identity confusion stemming
    from conflicting views of oneself as a successful abstainer vs. re-
    lapsed user.
(5) Feeling embarrassed and guilty about having let other people
    down, including family, friends, therapist, peers, etc.
(6) Feeling hopeless and helpless about staying off cocaine.

Since these feelings are a major contributor to precipitous dropout from
treatment, patients must be warned about them and taught how to cope.
One patient described it as follows:

When I slipped, I felt totally defeated, demoralized, and guilty. I
couldn't face anyone, not even myself. I didn't want to see my girlfriend,
go to group, or see my therapist. I wanted to crawl under a rock and
hide — with my freebase pipe. I thought my recovery was finished, blown
completely. I thought that the other group members wouldn't want to see
or talk to me anymore. These thoughts and fantasies just fueled my
continuing binge. The way I was looking at it — if I had lost everything
already, I had nothing more to lose by taking my drug use to the absolute
limit. I did more cocaine on that binge than I had ever used at one time
before. I wish that I could have kept it in perspective and dealt with it
better. I would have been a lot easier on me to look at it as a mistake, not
as the end of the world.

These feelings of failure can generalize and spill over into other areas of
the patient's life, compounding the problem, as described by another
patient:

I felt miserable about myself after I slipped, and I did it a number of
times. I was always so ashamed and embarrassed. I got to feeling that I
just couldn't trust myself. It was a profound and disturbing feeling, not

just a fleeting thought. And I would carry it into other areas of my life. I would feel bad about myself in every way imaginable. I got to the point of feeling that I couldn't do anything right, not a single damn thing.

IMPULSIVE ACTIONS

Abrupt, poorly thought-out, impulsive decisions and actions can sometimes precipitate relapse. In a fit of anger or frustration, the patient may quit his/her job, end a long-standing relationship, start an affair, drop out of treatment, stop attending self-help meetings, make an impulsive financial decision or investment. Often these hasty decisions have serious consequences that stimulate intense cravings for drugs.

ADDICTIVE AND COMPULSIVE BEHAVIORS

Related to impulsive actions are addictive and compulsive behaviors. These may be closely connected with previous cocaine use or emerge for the first time after the patient stops using drugs. As discussed in Chapter 6, many cocaine addicts have other addictions; the most common ones involve sex, gambling, spending, love relationships, food, and work. All addictions represent pathological relationships with a mood-altering experience, substance, or activity that is utilized to the point where it causes problems and adversely influences the quality of a person's life. They pose a threat to the person's well-being and to his/her abstinence from cocaine. Moreover, involvement in one addictive behavior often sets off desires to engage in other addictive behaviors. Continually opting for addictive "solutions" of any kind stalls recovery and makes continued abstinence from cocaine extremely difficult.

CO-DEPENDENT BEHAVIOR

Many cocaine addicts are also co-dependents who characteristically get caught up in the problems of others and give insufficient priority to addressing their own problems. This is particularly evident in patients who have been raised in families with parental addiction problems and/or those whose mates are also addicts. (It is not uncommon for adult children of addicts/alcoholics both to become addicts themselves and to choose other addicts as mates.) Co-dependent addicts are especially prone to "working someone else's recovery program" without working their own. In group sessions, they may make insightful comments and offer sound, enthusiastic advice to peers, but typically call very little attention to their own problems and share very little about their own personal feelings. Their attention and energy are always focused on someone else instead of themselves—an obvious, but usually unconscious defensive strategy that can quickly lead the patient in ιhe direction of relapse. The relapse progression is automatically set in motion by the absence of an active recovery program.

LETTING UP ON DISCIPLINES

Early relapse warning signs include lateness, sporadic attendance, and diminished involvement at group or self-help meetings, deviating from planned schedules, and balking at making a long-term commitment to re- covery activities — all of which can be seen as acting-out ambivalence about giving up the use of cocaine. Some patients are especially prone to "corner- cutting" when they feel that things are going well. This usually starts with small changes in behavior (e.g., coming only a few minutes late for meet- ings, not raising problems for discussion until the meeting is almost over and there is little time to discuss them), but can rapidly lead to a complete collapse in the patient's recovery program and a relapse to drugs. Silence is often an early warning sign: Patients who suddenly fall silent in group sessions or fail to say very much to begin with are almost always "sitting" on negative or self-defeating feelings that can derail their recovery plan.

Other Relapse Factors

UNTREATED PSYCHIATRIC DISORDERS

Cocaine addiction may be accompanied by coexisting psychiatric illness, especially mood and anxiety disorders which are primary problems and not merely byproducts of the chronic drug use. If left untreated, these disorders can impair thinking, moods, and behavior, create unacceptably high levels of stress, and thereby heighten the patient's potential for relapse. Patients who experience persistent dysphoria and other negative moods states despite con- tinued abstinence from drugs (especially those with a previous history of such disturbances prior to cocaine abuse) are prone to self-medicating these prob- lems with cocaine. Patients with severe narcissistic and borderline personality disorders also tend to be extraordinarily relapse prone as a result of their fragile self-esteem and difficulty in responding adaptively to painful affects.

MAJOR LIFE EVENTS

Major life changes — particularly negative, unexpected, and involuntary ones — create severe stress that can cause relapse. These changes may include the loss of a relationship, loss of a job, death of a loved one, or a sudden financial crisis. Also included are presumably "positive" changes which cre- ate a different kind of stress. For example, a job promotion may simultane- ously give the patient increased "disposable" income and increased responsi- bilities — both of which can increase temptations to use cocaine. Similarly, the birth of a child is usually a joyous event, but it also leads to increased responsibilities, reduced freedoms, and significant changes in the dynamics of existing family and/or marital relationships. Getting too quickly involved in a new intimate relationship early in recovery can also pose problems. Such "instant romances" typically result in profound disappointment and anger when the patient's unrealistic expectations are unmet.

PHYSICAL ILLNESS AND FATIGUE

Being physically ill, tired, or unfit can reduce the patient's coping abilities and increase his/her vulnerability to relapse. The AA slogan "H.A.L.T." (hungry, angry, lonely, tired) serves to remind recovering addicts of potential relapse danger signs. Neglecting one's health and physical needs, including the need for proper exercise, rest, and nutrition, can be indicative an overall lack of sufficient self-care to carry the patient through recovery.

FAMILY AND/OR THERAPIST ENABLING

Sometimes well-intentioned family members, therapists, and significant others enable or facilitate the patient's potential for relapse when they fail to set appropriate limits, ignore relapse warning signs, shield the patient from negative consequences of the addiction, and/or rationalize the patient's self-destructive behavior with psychological explanations and excuses. Patients who know by previous experience that significant others will rescue and shield them from the consequences of relapse are more likely to do just that — relapse.

RELAPSE PREVENTION STRATEGIES

Relapse can be prevented, but there is no simple and easy way to do it. Prevention strategies may be said to encompass any and all therapeutic measures that help a recovering addict avoid relapse, including virtually all efforts at treatment and self-help after initial abstinence is achieved.

While nonspecific measures such as individual psychotherapy may help to improve the addict's overall functioning and thereby reduce the possibility of relapse, the relapse prevention techniques discussed below represent intervention strategies that target specific risk factors and predictable features of the relapse process.

Relapse Prevention Group

A treatment group that focuses primarily and intensively on relapse prevention provides an effective forum in which patients can learn and apply principles of relapse prevention and recovery. The 16-week relapse prevention phase of our outpatient program includes a twice weekly group that combines intensive education and counseling focusing on relapse prevention and other drug-related issues. This is supplemented with individual and family counseling sessions.

The group format, as discussed more fully in Chapter 9 is uniquely effective in helping patients to recognize and overcome the obstacles to maintaining abstinence during the first few months of recovery. A relapse prevention workbook with writing exercises and checklists is used to help structure group discussions and review relevant issues as well as an educational video tape "Staying Off Cocaine" (Reelizations, Woodstock, N.Y.). The group provides patients with support, caring, and a sense of being part of a "team" whose major goal is to jointly maintain abstinence and prevent relapse. It also provides an opportunity for honest, immediate feedback and gentle, not heavy-handed, confrontation from peers in a way that penetrates the patient's denial and mobilizes adaptive problem-solving and coping skills.

Relapse Education

It is impossible to prevent something from happening if you don't know what to look for or how to handle it when it occurs. Patients are taught all of the concepts discussed so far in this chapter, including the definition of relapse, relapse myths, the relapse chain, relapse warning signs, relapse attitudes, and relapse behaviors, as well as how to recognize and deal with them. It is essential that relapse education be anchored to current experiences in patients' lives rather than presented in a purely didactic or academic fashion. While the 16-week group incorporates a specified sequence of lectures and discussion topics, this does not prevent the group from focusing on members' problems and issues as they arise. Often problems raised spontaneously by patients can be helpfully related to the topic under discussion and may even provide an opportunity to amplify and extend relapse education. Flexibility is the rule.

Admission vs. Acceptance

Part of preventing relapse is helping patients go beyond an intellectual admission that their addiction exists to a deeper, internal acceptance of the problem and its implications. This is an extremely critical task, the success of which may well determine whether or not relapse prevention strategies (or for that matter, any other treatment efforts) get through to patients in a way that produces lasting change.

When patients first enter the group, they often verbally and intellectually admit that they have a problem with cocaine, but usually do so with a good deal of reluctance and ambivalence. Although this admission is an essential beginning, it is insufficient for maintaining abstinence over the long term. Patients' continued ambivalence is inevitably acted out, and thereby revealed, as they fail to follow through on certain aspects of their recovery plan and discrepancies arise between what they say and what they actually do. Patients may intellectually understand the relapse process and relapse prevention strategies, but not fully accept the relevance of them to their own situation and as a result not fully apply them. Relapse education, no matter how complete or skillfully presented, may fall on deaf ears.

Therapeutic work within the group must focus on moving patients from intellectual admission to experiential acceptance of their inability to control drug use and their tendencies toward addictive thinking and self-defeating behaviors. Sometimes the patient's wall of defensiveness is not easily penetrated and genuine acceptance starts only when his/her attitude is transformed by a "conversion experience"—some type of consequence or event that stimulates a new, more adaptive way of looking at the addiction problem. Some patients show a significant attitude change after being confronted with a serious delayed consequence of their addiction (such as the loss of a relationship or job) or when they experience an actual slip or relapse due to an unsuccessful attempt at "controlled" drug use.

With acceptance comes greater openness, sharing, and willingness to utilize relapse prevention strategies and other tools of recovery. The patient demonstrates a stronger and more genuine commitment to maintaining abstinence, which is translated into actual behavioral and lifestyle change. Superficial, half-hearted compliance is replaced by willingness and even eagerness to work the program. The patient lets go of the need to control drug use, as well as the defiance and grandiosity associated with this need, and accepts help with gratitude rather than resentment. In short, the patient no longer fights the identity of being an addict in early recovery. The energy previously used in a self-defeating way to resist this identity is now channeled into adaptive problem-solving and coping strategies.

Self-Monitoring

Learning how to self-monitor thoughts, feelings, moods, behavior, and attitudes is an important skill for preventing relapse. Patients must become aware of the presence of relapse warning signs and risk factors before being able to respond to them appropriately. Self-observation skills can be acquired most easily in group settings, which provide opportunities to learn by imitation and feedback. Completing a weekly self-administered checklist or inventory of possible relapse factors, such as the one presented in Table 8.1, helps to increase the patient's awareness of relapse warning signs. A more extensive "Relapse Attitude Inventory," which is administered less frequently, is provided in Appendix G.

TABLE 8.1
Relapse Checklist

Negative Moods

Angry   Guilty
Depressed   Bored
Anxious, nervous   Tired
Lonely   Hungry
Sexually frustrated

Relapse Thoughts, Feelings, and Attitudes

Urges and cravings   Fantasies about controlled use
Impatience   Feeling sorry for myself
Overconfidence   Feeling hopeless
Expecting too much from others   Romanticizing the "good times" on
Blaming others   cocaine
Defiance   Feeling good and like celebrating with
Argumentativeness   cocaine
Defensiveness   Feeling hassled and justified in getting
Intolerance   high
Dissatisfaction   Feeling plagued by painful memories
Desire to test control   Feeling resentful toward others
Desire to indulge   Having drug dreams
Feeling like giving up   Wanting "magical" solutions to
Feeling unable to have fun without drugs   problems
Feeling elated—that everything is   Thoughts of dropping out
  "just fine"   of treatment
Feeling invulnerable to relapse   Dwelling on past mistakes
Doubting that I'm really an addict

Relapse Behaviors

"Backdoor setups": being in high-risk   Failure to take care of physical/medical
  situations   problems
Impulsive decisions or actions   Loss of daily structure
Other addictive/compulsive behaviors   Allowing stress and crises to build
Working someone else's recovery   Poor eating habits
  program   Lying
Coming late to meetings/sessions   Rejecting help
Missing meetings/sessions   Focusing on someone else's problems
Involvement in a new relationship too   instead of my own
  deeply, too soon   Becoming socially isolated, distant, and
Failure to exercise   withdrawn
Failure to plan leisure activities   Remaining silent

Ugly Reminders

An effective way to help patients counteract their tendency to idealize the cocaine high is encouraging them to keep visible reminders around of the negative consequences. For example, one patient was advised not to repair the damaged fender on his new car, the result of a cocaine-related accident, until he completed at least six months of abstinence. He described the benefits of this ugly reminder as follows:

At first, I didn't want to agree to it. I had worked so hard to get that beautiful machine, but now it seemed ruined by an ugly crumpled fender. I wanted to erase the memory as quickly as possible. But during the first few months of the program it helped me to see that twisted fender, especially when I had been daydreaming about the great times on cocaine. Seeing the fender set me straight — it let me know time and again that I couldn't have the pleasure of cocaine without the down side. There was the evidence, staring me right in the face.

Patients are also advised to make a running list of all cocaine-related consequences and a list of the reasons why they wanted to or were forced to quit in the first place. They are encouraged to refer to these lists whenever they find themselves romanticizing the high and/or experiencing active cravings or urges for cocaine. It is essential to teach patients how to "think through" the high — that is, how to take their thoughts beyond the high into the crash, the aftermath, the consequences, the guilt, and the disappointment — as a way of counteracting their selective recall and reducing the allure of cocaine. Patients are also encouraged to have a dramatically negative cocaine-related memory that they can "call up" to counteract euphoric recall, as described in the following three statements, each from a different patient:

When I'm actively caught up in glorified fantasies about cocaine, I have to go back to the worst possible moment I can remember on the drug — seeing a subway train coming into the station and thinking about throwing myself in front of it.

As soon as I start romanticizing the high, I think of my rent eviction notice, the harassing calls from bill collectors, not having enough money to put gas in my car.

I try to remember the terror, the times when I put myself in danger of being hurt, of having guys threaten to beat me up because I couldn't get some coke for them. Or the times when I was sick and had no one to help me. Those are the nightmares I try to keep fresh in my mind.

Relapse Scenarios

Having patients imagine and describe likely relapse scenarios is one of the best ways to help them anticipate and prepare for high-risk situations. Patients are asked to describe step-by-step exactly how the situation would come about, where and with whom, what feelings would be elicited, and what options would be available for avoiding relapse. Reviewing previous relapse episodes in this manner, including a detailed retrospective analysis of early warning signs and risk factors (facilitated by the Relapse Checklist), can be especially useful and revealing when patients have difficulty even imagining how they might ever relapse.

Updating Plans for Handling Cravings and Urges

Renewed cravings and urges for cocaine after a period of stabilization and abstinence require definitive action. Advance planning is crucial. Exactly how patients plan to respond to cravings needs periodic revisions, reminders, and updating. The handout in Table 8.2 can be helpful.

Cognitive Reframing

Correcting certain cognitive distortions or "mind traps" that generate maladaptive feelings and behaviors is an essential part of relapse prevention strategies. These self-defeating responses may include the patients' tendency to (a) overgeneralize or carry the implications of certain situations to an extreme; (b) take excessive personal responsibility for problems and mistakes beyond their control; (c) worry excessively and unnecessarily about antici-

---

TABLE 8.2
Points to Remember When You Have the Urge to Get High

1. Don't dwell on the pleasant memories of cocaine. Call up a negative memory or ugly reminder. Remember the aftermath of the last time you used cocaine. Think through the high.
2. Don't fall into the self-pity trap. None of your current problems will be solved or improved by using cocaine. They will only get worse.
3. Don't give up so easily. You have options. You have alternatives. Use them.
4. Call someone in your relapse prevention group. He/she will understand your feelings and help you out of them without using drugs.
5. Make an updated list of high-risk situations that could jeopardize your abstinence.
6. Make an updated list of your current support system.
7. Describe your current "emergency" plan.

pated problems; (d) see things in dichotomous, black-and-white terms; and (e) maintain a perfectionistic attitude toward recovery and react to any "rough spot" as indicative of personal weakness and failure. Cognitive restructuring techniques allow patients to reframe problems in ways that lead to potential solutions. The goal is to replace addictive thinking with basic problem-solving skills and adaptive coping strategies.

Stress Reduction

Excessive stress can disrupt the patient's functioning and initiate the relapse chain. Factors that contribute to high levels of stress include the following: taking on too many responsibilities; workaholism; trying to control and do everything oneself; poor communication with family, friends, and significant others; being overly competitive; being perfectionistic; being unable to "let go"; poor nutrition; lack of exercise; being too serious and lacking a sense of humor; excessive worrying.

Reducing stress usually requires that patients make significant changes in their lifestyle and daily routines. The first step is to help them identify the specific sources of stress and its negative effects on their attitude, mood, and behavior. Stress-reduction techniques include: exercise, sports, hobbies, and other leisure time activities; giving up caffeine and other artificial stimulants; practicing mediation, muscle relaxation, and biofeedback; delegating responsibility; getting organized at home and at work; avoiding procrastination and "quick fix" solutions; getting proper rest and nutrition; establishing routines and sticking to them; talking to friends about feelings and problems; making new friends; taking day trips on weekends; and taking periodic vacations.

Anger Management

Addicts commonly have problems in dealing with anger. Their anger is often disproportionate to the situation that provokes it. The feelings are ignored, displaced, suppressed, or sometimes acted out through the use of drugs or aggressive confrontations with others. Sometimes the anger is pent-up inside, causing passive-aggressive behavior and somatic symptoms such as headaches and ulcers. The people or situations that are the precipitants of the anger are avoided rather than dealt with appropriately. Table 8.3 includes steps suggested for handling anger effectively.

HANDLING RELAPSES

Managing a relapse successfully can be a difficult "tightrope walk" for the clinician. Patients typically feel embarrassed, disappointed, and angry when they relapse. They are exquisitely sensitive to any perceived rejection

TABLE 8.3
Steps for Handling Anger Effectively

1. Learn how to recognize the physical and psychological signs of angry feelings—muscle tension, clenched teeth, facial grimaces, irritability, short temper, nervousness.
2. Locate the sources of your anger. Examine recent situations and events. Are you angry at yourself or at someone else? Is your anger justified? Are you magnifying the problem or otherwise unnecessarily fueling your anger with irrational thoughts and expectations? Are you allowing the anger to build up to a boiling point?
3. Explore available options for handling your anger effectively. Talk to a third party. Discuss the issue with the person you're angry at, but only after you've calmed down and taken the opportunity to reflect on it rationally. Channel your anger into constructive activities—exercise, completing a project at home or at work, developing strategies to turn the situation to your advantage.
4. The next time you get angry, remember what worked for you the last time around. Remember that the feelings are temporary. No matter how uncomfortable they are right now, they do go away. Acting impulsively or exploding will just make everything worse.

or disappointment by others, particularly the therapist. The therapist's attitude and stance can strongly influence whether patients terminate their relapse or terminate treatment.

Therapists who respond to relapses as willful noncompliance and communicate negative attitudes of rejection, frustration, or hostility are likely to do more harm than good to relapsed patients. Such attitudes only confirm for the patients the destructive relapse myths mentioned earlier and provide them with further self-defeating justifications for continuing the relapse.

The relapse should be handled firmly and directly through gentle confrontation. An attitude of curiosity, concern, empathy, and understanding helps to reduce the patient's defensiveness and make him/her more amenable to examining the relapse episode in a clinically useful way. The therapist must not refrain from showing empathy out of fear that it will inadvertently condone the relapse and thereby promote future relapses. Being rejecting, punitive, or withholding is much more likely to do just that. Meanwhile, the therapist must not skirt, downplay, or give short shrift to the relapse.

Patients often fail to call or show up for their next counseling session after a relapse. They are reluctant to face their counselor or group after "failing" again. A timely call from the counselor or therapist communicating nonjudgmental concern and a genuine desire to explore what happened can begin to reverse the patient's downward spiral.

The goal is to set up a one-on-one relapse "debriefing" session as soon as possible after the relapse occurs, preferably before the patient returns to the group (but not while the patient is still intoxicated or crashing). The patient is reassured that the clinician has not given up on him/her. The relapse is reframed as an avoidable mistake rather than a tragedy. The patient is helped to recount, in detail, the events leading up to the relapse and to identify what warning signs were present. Suggestions are offered for dealing with the negative thoughts and feelings caused by the relapse. The patient is helped to identify specific steps that can be taken to avoid future relapses in the event that a similar set of circumstances recurs. Perhaps most importantly, revisions in the patient's treatment plan are discussed. For example, the patient may be encouraged to attend more self-help meetings, to attend individual and/or group sessions on a daily basis if needed until he/she has restabilized, to establish closer ties (through phone calls and socializing) with recovering peers, and generally to make better use of the treatment program.

The following is a brief segment taken from the beginning of a relapse debriefing session:

PATIENT   I guess I really blew it this time. I'm not sure that I can continue in the program. Nothing seems to work for me. I keep trying, but nothing changes. I didn't even enjoy myself. I felt horrible guilty and depressed from the very first snort. And the crash was even worse. Just when I thought I was doing OK—wham! I really thought I was working the program this time. I like the people in my group, I get a lot out of my sessions with you. I suppose you're pretty disappointed with me, and I bet the people in the group are too. I really let everyone down. Four months of being straight, right out the window. I don't know if I can start all over again. What's the use in trying—it'll just happen again anyway. Isn't that what it means to be an addict? You just keep relapsing and you just can't stop it, time and time again?

THERAPIST   It sounds like you're really feeling defeated by this whole thing, like all your progress up to now is lost, like you're helpless, hopeless, and that you should just give up. I don't see it that way at all. I think we can use this experience to help you avoid having another relapse. It's not a prophecy of doom or failure. You were doing pretty well for a long while and the progress you made is not lost. You can build on it, if you want to, or you can just throw up your hands and give up. I'm confident we can turn things around for you, if we both put our best effort into trying to figure out what happened and how to prevent it from happening again.

So you made a mistake. Maybe you just weren't paying enough attention to warning signs. Let's review exactly what happened, how you ended up getting high. If you recall, only a few weeks ago in the group we talked about exactly the type of defeatist reaction you're having right now and how relapse starts long before you actually get high again. I'm pretty sure that if we take a close look at what led up to your cocaine use, we'll find some valuable clues. We'll see that you were on the relapse track for quite a while, even though it feels to you right at this moment that it happened unexpectedly and completely out of the blue. My interest in you and my willingness to help you haven't changed a bit just because you've had a relapse. It's better not to have relapses if you can avoid them, but since it's already happened and we can't undo the past, let's not lose this opportunity to use it to your advantage. Describe to me as best you can exactly what happened. Don't try to analyze it yet, just stick as closely as you can to describing the sequence of feelings and events.

BEYOND RELAPSE PREVENTION

Treatment of the cocaine addict must never lose sight of the patient's potential for relapse — no matter how long patients have been abstinent or how motivated and stable they appear to be. Relapse vulnerability diminishes over the course of recovery, but never disappears entirely. It is permanent and lifelong — an immutable feature of addictive disease.

Beyond the specific relapse prevention strategies discussed above, what can be done to lower relapse potential over the long term? Lasting recovery requires significant changes in lifestyle, behavior, attitude, values, and personality. Addicts must change the way in which they solve problems, relate to others, think of themselves, and order priorities.

During the later stages of treatment, when abstinence is firmly established and relapse potential is markedly reduced, patients may benefit from psychotherapeutic approaches that are effective with non-addicts. Patients who complete the relapse prevention program are given the option of participating in an open-ended advanced recovery program, which offers individual and/or group psychotherapy and addresses patients' "addictive personality" along with other psychological problems, whether addiction-related or not. Patients are strongly encouraged to simultaneously continue their participation in self-help programs such as Cocaine Anonymous. Insight-oriented, supportive, directive, cognitive, and behavioral techniques are all utilized in order to "customize" the treatment to meet patients' individual needs.

A strong therapeutic alliance with the patient, coupled with mutual liking and respect, strengthens the possibilities for bringing about meaningful change. Nevertheless, no matter how stable the patient may be, anxiety generated during the psychotherapy process has the potential for precipitating relapse, so the therapist must always be mindful of this danger and immediately address the patient's increased relapse potential whenever it may occur.

Some of the treatment goals of this phase involve learning:

(1) To recognize and accept the full spectrum of one's feelings.
(2) To accept responsibility for one's behavior without self-blame.
(3) To manage flare-up periods without resorting to use of drugs.
(4) To overcome and grow beyond the arrested maturity and frozen development caused by chronic drug use.
(5) To manage uncomfortable or painful feelings adaptively, without acting-out.
(6) To make adaptive decisions and to take responsibility for those decisions.
(7) To have patience and to tolerate delayed gratification.
(8) To be honest, with oneself and others.
(9) To accept and view oneself realistically.
(10) To handle difficult, conflictual situations in an adult, self-satisfying manner.
(11) To accept and handle setbacks without having one's functioning deteriorate.
(12) To apply alternative coping strategies to handle feelings that were formerly self-medicated with drugs.
(13) To relate meaningfully to others.
(14) To have fun without drugs and to engage spontaneously in new, healthy activities.
(15) To let go of the past and to live more comfortably in the present.

CHAPTER 9

Group Therapy

GROUP THERAPY IS the core of outpatient treatment for cocaine addicts. It is perhaps the most potent and effective therapeutic modality for treating cocaine addiction and the best modality for applying most of the treatment strategies described in preceding chapters. Integrating the cocaine addict into a beginning recovery group is a first and critically important goal of outpatient treatment. Continued participation in group therapy through the early, middle, and later stages of recovery is often crucial to long-term treatment success. The rationale for the emphasis on group therapy and its unique advantages (as compared to individual therapy and self-help) are discussed in this chapter, along with practical issues pertaining to the clinical management of groups.

WHY GROUP THERAPY?

Group therapy is the most effective way to counteract the patterns of addictive thinking and behavior typically seen in addicts, especially cocaine addicts. Addiction is a disease of denial, deception, and delusion. It also leads to isolation, shame, and impaired social functioning. Cocaine addicts, especially those with pre-addiction histories of good functioning, frequently enter treatment with severely distorted ideas about themselves and the severity of their problem, issues that are dealt with very effectively in groups. Generally, they tend to overestimate their personal strengths and underestimate their vulnerabilities. It can be especially difficult for these patients to accept the concept of powerlessness over cocaine and the need to rely on others in order to overcome the problem. Even harder for them to accept is the notion that they have a lifelong addictive disease for which there is only recovery and no permanent cure.

Narcissistic personality disorders are common among cocaine addicts and, while many express strong desires for self-sufficiency, they nonetheless maintain strong emotional dependencies on others. They are apt to become very angry and disappointed when their excessive needs and demands are not instantly met. Deep-seated feelings of powerlessness and low self-worth are often masked by opposing outward defenses of manipulativeness, exploitive use of others, and a grandiose sense of self-importance and entitlement. The reality-testing, confrontation, and social support provided by groups are powerful tools for addressing these problems. It is extraordinarily difficult to deal with these types of behavior and feelings in individual therapy alone.

The Therapeutic Power of Groups

Enormous power is generated in groups that offer the combined input of treatment professionals and recovering peers. Such groups provide the support, role-modeling, reality-testing, and caring confrontation required to move patients through the myriad of obstacles in their lives and within themselves. Defensive roadblocks such as resistance, denial, and negative attitudes can fall away before recovering peers who share similar experiences. There is added credibility when the input of a "straight" professional is corroborated and expanded by the patient's peers. Group therapy serves as a multitude of unique therapeutic functions. Major among them are the following:

(1) mutual identification, acceptance, role-modeling, and confrontation;
(2) reality testing and immediate feedback;
(3) positive peer pressure;
(4) affiliation, cohesiveness, and social support;
(5) structure, discipline, and limit-setting;
(6) experiential learning and exchange of factual information;
(7) instillation of optimism and hope;
(8) pursuit of shared ideals.

Educational Function of Groups

Small groups are perfect for introducing educational components into the treatment program. For example, in our intensive program at least one or two meetings per week are begun with a brief topic-oriented lecture, film, or reading/writing assignment that delivers factual information and serves as a catalyst for group discussion. Topics include: understanding addictive disease; managing cravings and urges; the pharmacology of cocaine and other addictive drugs; the medical and psychological consequences of cocaine addiction; identifying high-risk situations; and the role of self-help in recovery. The group leader uses the discussion period afterward to personalize the material and help group members integrate this new learning into their own recovery.

Benefits to the Program

In addition to uniquely benefiting patients, group therapy has numerous advantages for the therapist and program as well. As compared to individual therapy, it is more time-efficient and cost-effective, a consideration especially important in many publicly funded clinics, where the demand for treatment often exceeds the capacity of the clinic's treatment staff. But apart from these practical considerations, group therapy offers unique opportunities for the therapist who also sees the patient individually (an optimal arrangement, in most cases) to observe a greater range of the patient's behavior, to see the reaction of others to the patient, and, perhaps even more importantly, to compare the patient's actual behavior with his/her self-perceived and self-reported behavior.

Groups also provide an excellent training ground, where aspiring group leaders have a chance to observe "live" role models in action while benefiting from experiential and didactic learning. Last but not least, groups are fun, stimulating, and rewarding. They provide a continuous source of learning for even the most experienced therapist.

GROUP THERAPY VS. SELF-HELP MEETINGS

Group therapy and self-help meetings are not good substitutes for one another. When used in combination, they enhance the cocaine addict's chances for successful recovery because each one complements the other.

Group therapy and self-help meetings differ from one another in significant ways. Groups are conducted under the leadership of a professional counselor or therapist, have limited membership prescreened by the group leader according to certain criteria, and are time-limited. Self-help meetings (such as Cocaine Anonymous), on the other hand, are conducted under the leadership of recovering peers who are simultaneously members of the group (reliance on treatment professionals is absolutely avoided and discouraged), have an unlimited membership with no prescreening of new members and no criteria for membership other than a desire to stop using drugs, and are open-ended (unlimited participation over the member's lifetime is not only possible but actively encouraged). Group therapy and self-help meetings share similar goals but utilize different strategies and address somewhat different needs. Because these important differences are not always clearly articulated or understood, many addicts and treatment professionals alike view these two forms of help as redundant or competitive, rather than complementary.

Benefits of Self-help Meetings

The unique benefits of self-help meetings result from their size, availability, and unified set of principles and beliefs designed to foster lasting abstinence and recovery from addictive disease. The large number of people usually present in self-help meetings promotes a powerful sense of belonging to a diverse community of peers. It provides members with a positive "subculture" that substitutes for a drug-using one and reduces the sense of loss that addicts typically experience when they give up their drug-oriented lifestyle.

Feelings of security, hope, and optimism are instilled by participating in a large support network that is engaged in the pursuit of shared ideals. The sense of unity, purpose, and shared identity engendered in self-help meetings is reflected in members' reference to outsiders (non-addicts) as "civilians"; members often relate to one another like "warriors" who are engaged in a common struggle against their disease. There is a sense of history, tradition, and continuity that is represented and reinforced by the presence of members who have been successfully recovering for many years. The diversity of membership in terms of sex, age, race, ethnicity, socioeconomic status, drug use history, etc., is a potent "equalizer" that promotes rapid identification and strong affiliative ties for newcomers. Feelings of uniqueness and shame are easily counteracted.

All self-help meetings are unified and empowered by the simple fact that they represent an assembly of fellow sufferers in high states of personal need who gather primarily to provide one another with a social support system and to share helpful advice. Other benefits include the following: a high level of availability (meetings are available throughout the day and evening, especially in large cities); the absence of membership fees (meetings are entirely self-supported through member donations—no outside funds are accepted); and the unconditional acceptance of new and returning members who need only show up and express a desire for help. All members, especially newcomers, are encouraged to link up with a "sponsor," an established member of the group who serves as an advisor, spiritual guide, and supportive friend. The sponsor's primary mission is to help other members utilize the self-help program as fully as possible and to foster his/her own recovery in the process of helping others.

Last but certainly not least, self-help programs are firmly anchored in a set of unified principles and beliefs (the 12 steps) designed to foster lifelong abstinence and promote physical, emotional, and spiritual well-being. An extensive self-help literature written specifically for and to the addict inspires hope and reinforces adherence to this belief system. The 12-step program incorporates several essential concepts and themes that are extraordinarily helpful to addicts:

(1) acceptance of addiction as a lifelong disease for which there is only recovery and not cure;
(2) the need for absolute abstinence from all mood-altering chemicals;
(3) the reliance on a "higher power" as a source of spiritual strength and guidance;
(4) the importance of addressing and resolving "character defects" as an integral part of the recovery process;
(5) the essential role of honesty, gratitude, and concern for others as cornerstones of recovery; and
(6) the importance of perseverance and active involvement in the self-help fellowship on a permanent, ongoing basis as the major vehicle for successful recovery.

Common Objections to Self-help

Despite the obvious benefits of attending self-help meetings, many cocaine addicts object to them and simply refuse to go. Common objections from patients are: "I'm not like those people at meetings, they're really sick and weird"; "I don't go for that spiritual nonsense, it sounds like religion to me"; "I don't think my problem is as serious as the people who go to those meetings, I don't think I really need to attend"; "Attending group therapy sessions is enough for me, I don't have the time or feel the need to go to meetings too."

By directly addressing these objections, the therapist can increase a patient's willingness to try self-help meetings and can also make sure that the patient isn't just inventing excuses for not having to put the effort into his/her recovery. Group therapy can be a very effective bridge to self-help. Group members who regularly attend self-help meetings often put pressure on those members who refuse to attend, challenging their reasons for avoiding self-help. They try to reduce some of the obstacles by offering to "escort" newcomers to a first meeting and to introduce them to others in the program.

Patients who strongly object to the program's mention of God, a "higher power," and other spiritual concepts may be told that neither adherence to any organized religion nor a belief in God is required to participate in self-help meetings. They can choose instead to make reference to any force or power greater than themselves that they are able to accept, such as forces of nature. Patients who overreact to this one aspect of the program are often looking for a way out.

Patients who complain that they don't identify with people at meetings should be encouraged to try a variety of different meetings until they do find a group of people with whom they can feel comfortable. The composition of meetings held at different times and locations, even within the same city or town, can vary greatly. Patients should be encouraged to sample at least a few different meetings before completely writing off the idea of becoming involved in self-help.

Lastly, when patients feel that a professional treatment program should be more than enough to resolve their cocaine addiction problem, they should be reminded that professional treatment is just the "launching pad" for recovery and is time-limited. Their addictive disease, however, is permanent, and unless they are actively involved in an ongoing program of recovery their relapse potential will remain unnecessarily high.

Benefits of Group Therapy

Group therapy derives its therapeutic potency from the clinical flexibility and intensity that only a small group conducted by a trained professional can provide. In addition to generating a strong sense of identity and belonging similar to self-help groups, small groups, with membership screened to insure homogeneity and balance, provide members with a unique opportunity for accelerated progress through guided feedback, continuity, role-modeling, peer pressure, didactic and experiential learning, and the acquisition of problem-solving skills. The group places high value on self-disclosure, active participation, compliance with group norms (e.g., abstinence, punctuality, attendance, honesty), and facing rather than avoiding problems.

It is difficult for resistant or non-interactive patients to "hide out" in small groups, as they sometimes do in large self-help meetings, since each member is the focus of attention for a while in every session. Acceptance by other group members is often based on a member's openness, sincerity, and demonstrated efforts to make positive behavioral change. Lying, "lip service," superficial involvement, and other signs of poor motivation are noticed and actively discouraged. The group is task-oriented and problem-oriented. It addresses important problems that contribute to or result from compulsive drug use. Common themes emerge in the group that serve as the focal point for group interaction, peer identification, and problem resolution. Advice, suggestions, and feedback provided by group leaders and other members help patients to develop self-monitoring skills and alternatives to drug use.

Senior group members share with newcomers advice and strategies that were helpful to them earlier in their own recovery. Similarly, newcomers provide the senior members with a chance to reflect on their own progress and at the same time supply helpful reminders about the chronic, insidious nature of addictive disease. Groups are an excellent way to orient and inform new patients about the treatment program, establish emotional equilibrium in early recovery, facilitate program retention and compliance as a by-product of bonding between members, and counteract emotional roadblocks to recovery as well as many of the unhelpful myths and misconceptions about cocaine use and recovery from cocaine addiction.

Small groups can be shaped to meet the differing needs of patients who are at different stages of recovery, as well as those who are grappling with special types of problems. For example, our outpatient program described in previous chapters offers a wide range of groups that address special needs including early abstinence groups, relapse prevention groups, advanced recovery groups, women's groups, men's groups, family groups, ACOA groups, and sexual addiction groups, each of which offers an opportunity to concentrate intensively on a particular set of issues or problems.

GROUP COMPOSITION

There is no pat formula for choosing the best mixture of patients for each group. Generally speaking, groups should be neither too heterogeneous nor too homogeneous with regard to members' age, gender, ethnicity, socioeconomic status, and educational background. Members who would be too extremely different from the others (e.g., one woman among all men, one gay among all heterosexuals, one psychiatrically disturbed person among all highly functional people) tend to feel out of place, drop out prematurely and inhibit the group's progress. There must be a good "fit" or good "chemistry" among group members, as well as a good fit between group members and group leaders. Newcomers find it easiest to integrate into an already formed group when they can readily identify with other members who share similar demographics and problems.

Cocaine addicts should be in groups with other cocaine addicts, but not necessarily in groups composed exclusively of cocaine addicts. Upon entering a group, newcomers tend to identify most readily with members whose drug histories are most similar to their own. In groups composed of cocaine addicts exclusively, route of administration often becomes a focal point for initial identification between group members. As relationships between members develop, similarity of drug histories becomes less important as a source of peer identification. It is preferable, wherever possible, to mix cocaine addicts with patients who are recovering from other types of chemical dependencies. Restricting group membership to cocaine addicts exclusively can be counterproductive: It tends to perpetuate an elitist attitude common among cocaine users and fosters an unhelpful notion that they are special people with unique problems.

When I first joined the group I could relate very well to the other freebasers in there whose problems sounded just like mine—the non-stop marathon binges for two or three days at a time, the paranoia, the horrible crash, the whole crazy scene. I was encouraged to see that people just like me had gotten past the cravings and were able to put down the pipe long enough to clear their heads up. It gave me hope. At first I didn't identify at all with the heroin addicts and alcoholics in the group. I was very judgmental about them: I thought the heroin addicts were a bunch of low-lifes and that the alcoholics were a bunch of lushes. I said to myself, 'I'm not as bad as them. I'm not in the street, I don't have to be here.' I thought that their problems would be totally different from mine, but the more I got to know them and hear their problems, the more I started seeing that we were all in the same boat. We had picked different drugs as our favorites, but we were all addicts. Our lives had became a mess because of our drugging and drinking. The problems and the pain were no different. Lots of our stories were interchangeable. We were more alike than different from one another even though some of us had 'front line' jobs and others were executive types. All of us had been cut down at the knees by drugs, whether we smoked them, snorted them, shot them, or drank them. We looked different on the outside—our outer shells were different—but inside our problems were pretty much the same.

Coed groups are the norm in the early and middle phases of treatment (i.e., in the intensive and the relapse prevention programs), although there are usually at least twice as many men as women in any given group due to the differing rates at which men and women enter addiction treatment.

Single-sex groups are utilized as adjuncts to the patient's primary recovery group in order to address special issues. Same-sex groups provide a safe atmosphere in which members can talk about sensitive or embarrassing problems (e.g., sexuality, relationship problems) that they normally avoid or do not feel comfortable discussing in coed groups. For example, female cocaine addicts who are struggling with guilt over having been promiscuous or having exchanged sexual favors for cocaine may be unable to talk about these issues in the company of men. Similarly, male cocaine addicts who have problems with sexual inadequacy or sexual compulsivity are often too embarrassed to mention these problems in the company of women.

Closed vs. Open Membership

Groups are limited in size to between eight and twelve members and routinely admit new members as others drop out. Because there is no way to guarantee that all members who start a group will actually finish it, open membership is a practical necessity in order to maintain an adequate membership for a viable group (usually six to eight members). When groups dwindle to fewer than six or seven members, it can become very difficult to maintain the morale and commitment of group members, because the survival of the group becomes tenuous and members fear that the group will dissolve if anyone else drops out.

There is always some initial discomfort and readjustment when new members join an ongoing group, but the potential benefits of open membership far outweigh the potential drawbacks. Newcomers at an earlier stage of recovery can derive immediate benefit from contact with the more advanced group members, who are often eager to take someone "under their wing." In this process, not only is the newcomer's learning and induction into the group accelerated, but the more senior member is given a chance to experience a greater sense of purpose and to receive additional feedback that marks his/her own progress.

Newcomers provide senior group members with vivid reminders of themselves at an earlier stage of recovery. Listening to newcomers helps to keep their memory "green"—to remind them of how unmanageable their lives had become on cocaine. This can counteract overconfidence, selective forgetting, and lingering fantasies about returning to controlled use. Additionally, the temporary shake up caused by the arrival of a new group member often has a positive impact on the progress of the group. New members add new points of view, new problems, new ideas, and a new set of life experiences, all of which can broaden the scope and effectiveness of the group experience for its members.

LEADERSHIP ROLES AND STYLE

Group leaders face many challenging tasks that determine the fate and effectiveness of the group. Among the leaders' most important functions are:

(1) To establish and enforce group rules in a caring, consistent, non-punitive manner to protect the group's integrity and progress;

(2) To screen, prepare, and orient potential group members to insure suitability and proper placement in the group;

(3) To keep group discussions focused on important issues and to do so in a way that maximizes the therapeutic benefit of these discussions to all members;

(4) To emphasize, promote, and maintain group cohesiveness and reduce feelings of personal alienation wherever possible;

(5) To create and maintain a caring, nonjudgmental, therapeutic climate in the group that both counteracts self-defeating attitudes and behaviors and promotes self-awareness, expression of feelings, honest self-disclosure, alternatives to drug use, and patterns of drug-free living;

(6) To handle problem members who are disruptive to the group in a timely and consistent manner to protect the membership and integrity of the group; and

(7) To educate patients about selected aspects of drug use, addiction, recovery, etc., as a way of transmitting potentially useful information and as a catalyst for group discussion.

Leadership style is determined by many factors, not the least of which are the leader's personality, theoretical orientation, and experience in running groups. Irrespective of these factors, effective leadership of a drug recovery group demands that the leader adopt a certain posture in the group that differs significantly from that in traditional psychotherapy groups. In the latter, the therapist gently guides and focuses the attention of group members on matters pertaining to group process, group dynamics, and the complicated interpersonal interaction among group members. With the exception of carefully timed comments, the therapist may remain passive, quiet, and nondirective in the customary mode of traditional psychotherapy.

By contrast, in drug recovery groups the therapist must be very active in keeping the group focused on concrete here-and-now issues that pertain directly to drug-related matters, especially in early abstinence groups. The therapist plays a very active and directive leadership role, which includes questioning, confronting, advising, and educating group members on relevant issues. He/she keeps the group task-oriented and reality-based and serves as the major catalyst for group discussion. Addressing addiction-related issues is always the number one priority of the group and the therapist must be sure to keep the group focused on that task.

Single vs. Co-leadership

Single leadership of recovery groups is stressful, difficult, and not nearly as effective as team or co-leadership. Co-leadership has numerous advantages, including shared responsibility by the two leaders for the supportive, confrontational, and administrative (management) tasks involved in running the group. Patients benefit from the dual input of two leaders. The presence of a second leader expands the options for interaction in the group and usually accelerates group progress. It also helps to diffuse intense anger and other negative feelings that patients may develop temporarily toward one or the other leader. It is more difficult to rationalize that both leaders are all wrong.

Despite its potential advantages, co-leadership, unless orchestrated properly, can cause serious problems in the workings of a group. This is likely to happen when group leaders are unfamiliar or overly competitive with one another, have clashing personalities and/or clinical styles, or fundamentally disagree about how the group should be run. Obviously, co-leaders must carefully assess their compatibility with one another and work out the details of their collaborative roles in the group before joining forces. Their efforts in the group must be complementary, synergistic, and cooperative. At the very least, the leaders should not differ significantly from one another in their basic views about addiction and recovery. Both must work comfortably within the disease model, and both must agree on the fundamental rules, purpose, goals, and membership criteria for the group. They must acknowledge differences that might arise and use them constructively to benefit the group. Patients should not be made to suffer from discord and competitiveness between group leaders. Poor coordination and communication between group leaders provides negative interpersonal role modeling, which is distinctly countertherapeutic and threatens the safety of the group in a way that is often very upsetting and detrimental to patients.

However, it is neither necessary nor desirable for co-leaders to agree with one another on every issue that comes up in the group. Differences in point of view, theoretical orientation, interpretation, and suggestions, when handled constructively, can substantially broaden the options made available to patients and greatly enhance the therapeutic power of the group. It can be very instructive and therapeutic for patients to see group leaders handling their differences constructively.

In order to maximize their collaborative functioning, group leaders must meet with one another regularly to discuss the group—the interaction among members and leaders, and the problems and progress of the group. They should allocate time, if possible, to debrief one another after each group session and to discuss strategies for the next session. They must also communicate relevant information to one another from contact with members outside group meetings, as in telephone calls and individual therapy sessions.

An optimal co-leadership team consists of a professional therapist (with extensive group therapy and addiction treatment experience) as the primary leader of the group and a recovering cocaine (or other drug) addict as the co-facilitator. The co-facilitator must be someone with at least two years of stable abstinence and solid recovery who has successfully "graduated" from previous group therapy and is meaningfully involved in a 12-step program of self-help, such as CA, AA, or NA (without this latter requirement the co-facilitator cannot serve as a credible role model for encouraging patients to become involved in self-help).

Among the unique benefits of having recovering addicts as co-facilitators is the greater credibility they usually enjoy on certain issues with patients as compared to "straight" professionals. They are sometimes better able to confront a group member's denial or other problems in a way that is less likely to elicit defensiveness, especially when they draw upon their own similar experiences at an earlier stage of recovery. They serve as "live" role models for recovery and progress in the group.

The role of the recovering addict co-facilitator is best described as being somewhere between that of a group leader and a group member. He/she may slide between these two poles as the needs of group members dictate. For example, in trying to confront a highly resistant and defensive group member, the co-facilitator may talk from the vantage point of a fellow addict who knows all too well what it feels like to be in that same frame of mind and what problems it can cause. The message communicated to the patient is one of peer identification and empathy: "I'm just like you. I have a tendency to think that way too. I know exactly how you feel." In other situations, the co-facilitator may speak more from the vantage point of a counselor offering feedback, advice, or encouragement. Here the co-facilitator is likely to draw on his/her own therapy experience, intuitive good sense, and supervision from the group leader. In this regard, it is essential that the group leader provide the co-facilitator with ongoing supervision outside of the group meetings.

Among the common but usually surmountable problems to be expected when recovering addicts serve as co-facilitators are tendencies: (1) to over-generalize from their own recovery and treatment experiences in a way that may leave patients feeling inadequately understood as individuals; (2) to become overly angry and frustrated with noncompliant patients and to sometimes act out this anger by harshly confronting them; and (3) to feel generalized discomfort or even active cravings and urges as a result of the group's intensive focus on drug-related issues. Before joining a group for the first time, co-facilitators should be made aware of these potential problems and encouraged to deal with them in supervisory sessions.

In addition to holding regular supervisory meetings, the group leader should allocate at least 15–20 minutes after each group session to debrief the co-facilitator, in order to diffuse any strong feelings stirred up in the group and to briefly review what took place in the session. Although co-facilitators sometimes find their participation in groups to be stressful, when handled appropriately it usually accelerates their own recovery by bringing to their attention important therapeutic issues.

Screening New Group Members

A vital function of the group leader is to serve as the "gatekeeper" of the group — to evaluate and screen prospective group members for suitability and placement in a group. The leader must protect the group's integrity, its goals, and its membership in order to maintain an atmosphere of safety, consistency, and therapeutic focus. Leaders who permit patients to enter the group without adequate screening may find the group demoralized as a result of having one or more problem members among them: people who are not "team players," who don't fit in well with the rest of the group, or who, because of disruptive behavior or lack of motivation, do not belong in the group at all.

Not all cocaine addicts are appropriate for group therapy. Some are too severely disturbed or anxiety-ridden to tolerate group treatment. Patients who suffer from extreme anxiety, paranoia, emotional lability, or other serious psychiatric problems should not be coerced into group treatment. Any such attempt could exacerbate these preexisting problems and lead to further deterioration in the patient's functioning — and damage the group as well. Some of these patients can be gradually phased into groups as a goal of early treatment, but only with intensive preparation on an individual basis.

Apart from the presence of serious functional impairment or psychiatric illness, it is often difficult to predict which cocaine addicts will do well in group therapy. The patient's actual behavior in early group sessions, which can be thought of as an extension of the evaluation process, usually indicates to what extent he/she can accept or be accepted by the group. Newcomers who exhibit destructive or disruptive behavior and those who are inordinately stressed or overwhelmed by the group are sometimes removed from it as quickly as possible to prevent them from experiencing adverse effects and to preserve the integrity of the group.

Many patients who could benefit from group treatment and are appropriate for it react negatively to the idea of entering a group. Common objections are: "I don't see any benefit in talking with a group of strangers about my personal problems or sitting there listening to their problems." "I'm a private person, I'm concerned about confidentiality, and I'd rather just talk to you alone in individual sessions." Patients most likely to object to groups are those who have been in lengthy individual analytically-oriented psychotherapy and those who have had bad experiences (such as harsh confrontation) in previous group therapy. In addition, cocaine addicts who are executives or professionals often have grave concerns about confidentiality and balk at the idea of entering a group.

Patients who object to group therapy are asked to try it for one week before making a final decision. Usually, their fears are dispelled when they meet others in the group who are very similar to themselves. Once the newcomer forms an initial bond with another group member, the chances that he/she will elect to continue in the group are greatly increased. Patients who are poorly motivated or disobey the basic group rules should not be put into groups, even temporarily. They tend to anger and demoralize other group members and derive little benefit from the experience. Group membership must be regarded as a privilege for newcomers and not a right, in order to preserve the integrity of the group.

PREPARING NEW MEMBERS FOR GROUP ENTRY

Patients must be prepared for group entry so that they begin with realistic goals and expectations. Before admitting new patients into the group, the leader should see them individually for a few days in order to assess motivation, clarify myths and misconceptions about group therapy, and address any resistance to group participation. Many patients have stereotyped images of groups as places where they will be harshly confronted, humiliated, and punished for "bad" behavior. Patients are educated about the purpose, goals, expectations, rules, composition, content, and format of the group as well as the respective roles of group members and group leaders. One strategy that is used to counteract initial resistance and fears about entering group treatment is to arrange a one-on-one meeting between a prospective new group member and one of the more senior members of the group who is willing to share his/her group experiences and answer questions.

A vital prerequisite to entering an early recovery (beginners') group is for prospective new members to achieve at least four or five days of abstinence immediately prior to attending their first group meeting. Not only does this give patients time to recover from the acute aftereffects of cocaine, but it also validates their motivation to become drug free and screens out those who may be unwilling or unable to stop using cocaine. Established group members are understandably intolerant of newcomers who are still actively using drugs or are only a day or two from their last high—they usually react with a mixture of disgust and jealousy. Active users are likely to spark intense cravings in group members who have been abstinent themselves for only a short while.

The basic ground rules and guidelines for group participation should be spelled out in writing and signed by each newcomer before entering the group (see Table 9.1).

HANDLING PEER CONFRONTATION

Peer confrontation is an extremely effective therapeutic tool in groups, but heavy-handed, excessive, and poorly timed confrontation can be countertherapeutic. Some patients enter groups with the mistaken idea that humiliation and aggressive confrontation are acceptable ways to force resistant

TABLE 9.1
Group Rules

1. I agree to come to group sessions completely "straight," not under the influence of any mood-altering chemicals whatsoever.
2. I agree to abstain from the use of alcohol and all drugs during my participation in the group.
3. I agree to attend all scheduled sessions and to arrive on time without fail. I will postpone all vacations and out-of-town trips while participating in the group.
4. I agree to preserve the anonymity and confidentiality of all group members. I will not divulge the identity of any group member or the content of any discussions to persons outside the group.
5. I agree to remain in the group for its stipulated duration. If I have an impulse or desire to leave the group prematurely, I will raise this issue for discussion in the group before acting on these feelings.
6. I agree to not become involved romantically, sexually, or financially with other group members for the duration of my participation in the group.
7. I agree to accept immediate termination from the program if I offer drugs or alcohol to any member of the group or use these substances together with any group member.
8. I agree to have my telephone number(s) added to the list distributed to all group members.
9. I agree to give a supervised urine sample at each group meeting and whenever the group leader may request it.
10. I agree to raise for discussion in the group any issue which threatens my own or another member's recovery. I will not keep secrets regarding another member's drug use or other destructive behavior.

TABLE 9.2
Guidelines for Successful Confrontation

1. Confrontation is defined as giving someone realistic feedback about their behavior as you see it. It is a process by which you attempt to "hold up a mirror" to let a person know how he/she appears to others. It is not an attempt at "character assassination."
2. Confrontation is most useful when spoken with empathy, concern, and caring in a respectful tone of voice.
3. Confrontation is descriptive of what you have observed, giving examples of the behavior in question. It excludes guesses, explanations, interpretations, advice, and criticisms about the person's behavior.
4. Confrontation includes a statement of your concern about the person's dangerous, self-defeating behavior and, if possible, an example of similar self-defeating behavior from your own experience.

members of the group to face reality. Sometimes harsh confrontations are rationalized as attempts to be "truly honest" with members who violate group expectations and norms. Group members typically have less tolerance for negative attitudes and "b.s." than do group leaders, especially when these attitudes are reminiscent of their own. Likely targets for attack are members who repeatedly relapse, who remain defiant, superficial, and insincere, and who minimize their problem and fail to genuinely affiliate with other members of the group.

Sometimes group leaders feel ambivalent about stopping attacks on group members with thorny problems that have long been overlooked. The group leader must never allow unpopular, frustrating, resistant, or severely troubled group members to be scapegoated and bludgeoned by their peers even when the content of what is being said is entirely accurate. Harsh or excessive confrontation must not be used as a means to push selected members out of the group or to discourage them from coming back.

It is the style rather than the content of peer confrontation that determines its impact on the designated group member. The main goal of confrontation is to make the person more receptive to change without eliciting defensiveness or destructive acting-out behavior. Table 9.2 lists guidelines we give patients on how to effectively confront their peers.

HANDLING PROBLEM GROUP MEMBERS

Certain group members may cause serious problems and disrupt the functioning of the group. For example, some members are chronically antagonistic, argumentative, volatile, and sarcastic. Even those who emphatically state how much they need the group may nonetheless take every opportunity to devalue the group, complain about how poorly it is run, point out even the most minor inconsistencies, and categorically reject advice or suggestions from members and leaders of the group. Problem patients may attempt to monopolize group sessions, feeling resentful or disrespectful of the time devoted to other members' problems and never feeling that enough time is devoted to their own problems.

Some problem patients are just the opposite: They sit silently in groups, glad to have the attention always focused on someone else. Silent members are often hiding intense feelings of ambivalence, resentment, anger, and fear. Often, patients who have slipped or run into serious or embarrassing problems, even if they were previously talkative in groups, may suddenly become silent and unresponsive—a clear outgrowth of addictive thinking that says, "If there's a problem, ignore it, pretend that it doesn't exist."

Patients who are chronically depressed and non-interactive in groups may also cause problems by casting a shadow of gloom and hopelessness over the group that stalls its movement. They may evoke uncomfortable feelings of pity and sorrow in other members who then avoid paying attention to them or act as if they did not exist.

Patients who come to groups while actively intoxicated or crashing from drugs (a very rare occurrence since being in a group session is probably the last place someone in either state would want to be) can cause havoc in the group. They must be asked to leave the session immediately.

The leader must vigilantly monitor and manage the behavior of problem group members and gauge their impact on the rest of the group. Sometimes the content of what patients say in group is less important than the way in which they say it. The leader must continuously attend to patients' affect and communication style. Sarcastic and aggressive statements should not be ignored or overlooked. Patients should not be allowed to monopolize the group with tirades or intellectualized discourses. When this occurs, the leader should ask other group members why they are permitting one member to take up so much of the group's time without interruption. Don't they have other important issues to discuss? If not, why not?

Silent members must also be confronted with their nonparticipation in the group. They must be helped to see how they are using their silence to avoid facing important issues and how silence is an enemy of their recovery. Severely depressed patients who are unable to interact in groups may require psychotropic medication or even hospitalization.

A special issue in managing problem patients is the formation of subgroups that undermine the group and sometimes threaten its very survival. Divisive members may work behind the scenes, chipping away at group cohesiveness, while simultaneously maintaining a façade of cooperativeness. They form ties with certain group members that intentionally exclude other members, causing a build-up of tension and hostility between different "factions" in the group. These subgroups can quickly strangle group interaction, bring the therapeutic movement of the group to a grinding halt, and precipitate dropouts. Certain members who had been active in the group may suddenly fall sullen and silent, and there may be a total absence of meaningful dialogue in group sessions. The leader is often the last to find out about the existence of these subgroups, since most members want to avoid being the person who "spills the beans."

Dangerously divisive group members who threaten the recovery of other members or the survival of the group itself should be expelled from the program immediately, as in the case of one patient who was secretly pressuring other group members to leave the treatment program and form a new "group" that would meet every week at his home. When he failed to show up at the group meeting, one of the patients he was pressuring revealed the sabotage plan. Group members then talked openly about their conflicting feelings and how these feelings were stimulating intense cravings for cocaine and fantasies about quitting treatment. Shortly thereafter, the divisive group member was confronted by the leader in a telephone conversation and told not to return to the group, much to the relief of other group members. He had severely relapsed to smoking freebase cocaine, was in a paranoid psychotic state, and flatly refused all offers of help.

Whenever problem patients seriously disrupt or stall the therapeutic movement of the group and remain chronically unresponsive to interventions by the group leader and fellow group members, they should be removed from the group, either temporarily or permanently. Sometimes temporary suspension from the group coupled with intensive individual therapy during an interim period can help to resolve some of the intense feelings or crises that may have been contributing to a patient's difficulty in the group. Group members are usually more relieved than upset when the leader takes decisive action with problem patients to preserve the safety and integrity of the group.

FACILITATING TRANSITIONS IN AND OUT OF GROUPS

In a treatment program that is divided into successive and discrete stages, each with its own goal-oriented groups, issues involving the transition of patients in and out of groups come up frequently. The most difficult transition for patients is usually their initial induction into the beginner's intensive group. This is especially true for patients who have had no prior group therapy experience and enter the group on the heels of active cocaine use. Having to deal all at once with the initial tasks of developing comfort, trust, and affiliation in the group can be overwhelming. Some newcomers respond very positively to attempts by existing group members to reach out to them.

Others recoil, preferring to maintain their distance until they decide whether or not they feel comfortable enough in the group to stay. Sometimes pushing a newcomer too hard to connect with other group members before he/she is really ready to do so can backfire and send him/her running away from the group. The leader's judgment and guidance here are crucial.

When patients "graduate" from one phase of the program to the next, every attempt is made to ease the transition by placing them into a group with the same group leader and with one or more patients from their previous group. Continuity of treatment is also assured by assigning patients to the same therapist for both individual and group therapy. To facilitate smoother transitions between groups, during the final three weeks of each treatment phase patients are actively encouraged to discuss their feelings about leaving the group. Most express ambivalence: They feel good about making progress and moving on to the next stage of recovery, but sad about leaving the group behind. They often experience anticipatory anxiety about what the next stage of treatment will bring. Will they have to get at the real "root" of their cocaine problem? How can they face some difficult realizations about themselves?

Not surprisingly, it is a time when patients commonly experience a temporary return of negative moods, cravings for cocaine, and a general increase in relapse potential. Knowledge of this phenomenon can prepare both the therapist and the patient to deal more effectively with the situation and to not respond in ways that only increase the patient's chances for a regressive relapse.

HANDLING SLIPS AND RELAPSES

Specific strategies for handling slips and relapses were discussed in Chapter 8, but the special problem of handling this issue in groups warrants separate discussion here. When group members report that they have used drugs since the last session or their urine test indicates that this is so, the group must give priority to addressing this issue. In addition to the expected feelings of embarrassment and guilt by those members who have slipped, all group members usually have strong feelings in response to another member's use of drugs. These must be aired.

Discussion of a group member's drug use generally proceeds as follows:

(1) The member who has slipped is asked to provide the group with a detailed account of the sequence of feelings, events, and circumstances that lead to the slip.
(2) Other group members are encouraged by the leader to further question the drug-using member, in a nonjudgmental way, about early

warning signs, self-sabotage, and other factors that may have preceded the drug use.

(3) The group leader summarizes and restates the relapse chain which appears to have led up to the patient's drug use.

(4) Group members arc asked to share any suggestions or feedback they can offer to the drug-using member about the slip and how to prevent it from happening again. They are also asked to share their feelings about the slip, but the group leader reminds them to avoid any tendency they may have to scapegoat the drug-using member or to act out feelings of anger and frustration on him/her.

(5) With the participation of the drug-using member, a list of suggested strategies and behavioral changes is developed to guard against the possibility of further drug use.

(6) The member who has slipped is asked to share his/her thoughts and feelings about what he/she has learned as a result of the slip and to describe his/her willingness to take action to reduce the chances of using drugs again.

Although most group members respond supportively to another member's slip, there is an unspecified limit as to how often drug-using members can expect this type of supportive response. When members have slips repeatedly, regularly, and show little or no evidence of utilizing the advice and suggestions offered by the group, others become intolerant and begin to feel that the group is enabling its drug-using member(s). This can happen after two slips, three slips, four slips, etc., depending on the overall attitude and behavior of the drug-using member and the nature of his/her relationships with others in the group. The decision to temporarily suspend a drug-using member from the group usually develops from the collective feelings and attitudes expressed by other group members in combination with the clinical judgment of the group's leaders. This type of decision-making process is preferable to specifying in advance exactly how many slips patients are allowed before they are suspended from the group. If, for example, patients were told at the outset that three slips would result in suspension, this would be tantamount to giving them permission to have up to two slips — a distinctly countertherapeutic message!

INTERFACE WITH INDIVIDUAL THERAPY

Although group therapy is the preferred modality of treatment for most cocaine addicts, it is usually insufficient by itself to address the full range of issues and problems experienced by those who enter treatment. A combination of individual and group therapy is optimal for most patients, preferably with the same therapist conducting both forms of treatment. When the patient's group leader also serves as his/her individual therapist, the usual problems in coordinating these two forms of treatment are eliminated. The dual role of the therapist provides an opportunity to directly observe a wider range of the patient's behavior first hand and to use the information obtained about the patient in one treatment context to maximize the effectiveness of interventions utilized in the other. For example, when patients actually display certain problems in group sessions that have been previously identified and discussed in individual sessions, the therapist has a unique opportunity to draw connections between the two. This type of interplay between individual and group therapy can have very potent synergistic effects, thereby accelerating the treatment and recovery process. Issues raised in group sessions often serve as catalysts for discussions in individual sessions and vice versa.

Individual therapy also gives patients an opportunity to address certain sensitive or embarrassing issues such as those involving intimate relationships, sexual functioning, business problems, and self-esteem. The therapist should not rigidly insist that patients discuss any and all personal matters in the group. Similarly, the therapist must guard against violating the patient's confidentiality on certain defined issues. It is essential that the patient and therapist clarify with one another exactly which issues discussed in individual therapy sessions are not to be mentioned in group sessions. However, issues directly involving the patient's drug use must be categorically excluded from any such agreement: The therapist's hands cannot be tied when it comes to dealing with drug-related issues in the group and there can be no secrets about drug use among group members.

When patients are referred for group treatment by an outside therapist who plans to continue seeing the patient in individual psychotherapy, the group leader must obtain the patient's permission to communicate with the individual therapist. When the two therapists communicate regularly and agree on a coordinated treatment plan, the two treatments can work well together. Both therapists must guard against the splitting defense of some patients (particularly those with narcissistic and/or borderline personality disorders), i.e., the patient's tendency to pit one therapist against the other in a way that deflects his/her personal responsibility for making change.

OUTSIDE CONTACT AMONG GROUP MEMBERS

Group members are actively encouraged to maintain contact with one another outside the group. (Again, this is very different from traditional psychotherapy, where outside contact among group members is viewed as an undesirable "contamination" of the group's therapeutic environment.) A list of telephone numbers of all group members, routinely updated when newcomers enter the group, is circulated to all members. In order to promote their rapid induction into the network of existing members and to foster group cohesiveness, newcomers are asked to call at least one group member every day during their first two weeks in the group. Members are encouraged to plan social activities together, to go with one another to self-help meetings, and to call one another in time of need. One of the most important functions of the group, especially for newcomers, is as a support network to interrupt cravings and urges to use cocaine. Patients are expected to report any contact they have had with one another between group sessions at the next meeting.

ATTENDANCE, LATENESS, FEES

Consistency and predictability are essential to group treatment. Members must attend regularly, the only exception being truly unavoidable or extreme circumstances. Since most patients have histories of being generally irresponsible and unreliable during their active addiction, they must not be allowed to continue this behavior in the group. The group leader must begin and end all group sessions on time. Members who are chronically late or absent and fail to change this behavior despite warnings from the leader and pressure from other group members may have to be expelled from the group. Chronic lateness and absenteeism are indicative of ambivalence about giving up cocaine and grow out of the patient's denial about whether or not he/she is really addicted to the drug and whether the problem is really serious enough to warrant treatment. When fees are charged, they must be paid on time. Patients who are allowed to build up large outstanding balances of unpaid fees almost invariably drop out of treatment precipitously and prematurely.

A well-organized and well-run group serves as an example to patients of how planning and consistent follow-through are essential to achieving desired goals. Patients are able to extrapolate from their experiences in a well-run group how to better organize and run their own lives—an essential goal of treatment. The group becomes a "learning laboratory" for acquiring basic life-management skills, including planning one's time, avoiding procrastination, dealing with unanticipated problems, and paying attention to the needs of others.

CHAPTER 10

Cocaine and the Family

When Kevin, a 17-year-old high school student, needed money to buy crack, he would steal it from his parent's dresser drawer, take the family car without permission, and disappear on a two-day binge. When he returned home, irritable and short-tempered from "crashing," his mother's inquiries about where he had been usually led to violent arguments. Kevin's parents tried to convince him to enter a treatment program, but he refused, saying that he didn't need anyone else's help. The parents were living in a state of terror and depression because of Kevin's problem. They were both suffering from insomnia and lack of adequate sleep from staying up at night trying to prevent Kevin from sneaking off to get high. They hadn't had sex for nearly eight months. Their social life had become nonexistent. Kevin's mother complained of frequent panic anxiety attacks; his father complained of migraine headaches. Although they wanted Kevin to stop using drugs, they continued to leave cash in predictable "hiding" places, fearing that he would commit a crime and perhaps be arrested if they didn't give him access to money when he was feeling desperate.

David, a 35-year-old businessman, had brought his marriage to the brink of disaster through cocaine addiction. At least once or twice a week he would leave home in the evening, supposedly to buy a pack of cigarettes or take a walk, and then not return home or call for two days. His cocaine binges involved marathon sex orgies with prostitutes in fancy hotel rooms. David's wife suspected that his cocaine use involved other women, but she nonetheless constantly "covered his tracks"—made excuses to his boss and others—in order to minimize the fallout from his irresponsible and erratic drug-induced behavior. She tried everything she knew in order to get David to stop using drugs: threats, blackmail, bribery, suicide gestures, calls to the police, and leaving with the kids for a day or two at a time. She felt inadequate as a wife, believing that if she were just sexier, prettier, more fun-loving herself David wouldn't be so inclined to use cocaine. She threatened numerous times to leave him permanently, file for divorce, and take their two young children with her, but David quickly learned that these were idle threats. She kept hoping that he would seek help, but the problem just continued to get worse. She became chronically depressed, lonely, and isolated. She hated having a "part-time" husband who seemed not to care enough about her or their children to stop using cocaine. She finally sought treatment, saying that she felt trapped in an impossible bind. She loved David and felt sorry for him, but knew that she had to do something to save herself and her children from this horrible mess.

Jean, a 29-year-old legal secretary, rarely had enough money to pay her rent, food, or clothing bills due to her chronic use of cocaine. She had been arrested once for dealing drugs and once for passing bad checks in order to get money for drugs. On both occasions her parents bailed her out of trouble. When Jean complained of being broke and depressed, her parents (knowing that she was using up her entire salary on drugs) would pay her rent, stock her refrigerator with food, and give her credit cards to buy new clothes. After Jean nearly died from an overdose of sleeping pills but still refused to enter a treatment program, her parents sought help for themselves. They knew that they were participating in a destructive relationship with Jean, but felt unable to stop.

Jean's mother, Ann, wanted immediately to stop giving her any more money. Her father, Bernard, on the other hand, simply couldn't accept the idea of totally "abandoning" Jean in that way—he refused to even discuss the matter even though he felt terrorized and held hostage by her drug problem. Bernard had suffered a heart attack two years before but failed to follow through on his doctor's orders to work less compulsively, spend more time involved in leisure activities, and lose weight by changing eating habits and attending an exercise program. Although he had planned to retire soon, he now felt increased financial pressures from having to support Jean and was unable seriously to think about his own life until Jean stopped using drugs and entered a program. He was obsessed with thoughts about Jean at work and at home, and often stayed up at night worrying about her. His wife was becoming increasingly angry at him for refusing to take action. While sitting at his desk at work, Bernard suffered a massive heart attack and died.

As seen in these case examples, cocaine addiction is a problem that often affects the entire family, sometimes in an extremely negative, even deadly, way. The impact of cocaine addiction on the family is not dissimilar to that of alcoholism. There are frequent arguments and severe problems as a result of the user's negative, changing, unpredictable moods as well as his/her erratic, irresponsible behavior, including unexplained absences and inability to function. Increasingly, the addict neglects responsibilities and withdraws from family activities, preferring to spend time getting high alone or with other drug users. If the addict is a spouse or parent, others in the family often experience profound loss and rejection. If the addict is a teenager who stays out at night and breaks curfews, parents usually become frustrated and angry at being unable to exert effective control. In any case, addicts often become increasingly defensive, hostile, and sometimes even violent when confronted with their irresponsible behavior. Their communication with the rest of the family all but completely shuts down.

But the most profound and damaging effects occur silently and insidiously, within individual members of the household, as they inevitably react to the chronic state of crisis and confusion. These changes are usually internal, subtle, barely perceptible at first. More and more, as the drug-related problems continue, family members' attention and energy shift from their own needs, interests, and concerns to those of the addict. The family's functioning comes to revolve around the problems of the addict: trying to figure out whether or not he/she is using drugs again; reacting to the addict's irrational behavior; searching for the addict's hidden drug supplies; monitoring the addict's telephone conversations; searching the addict's belongings; pleading and fighting about the addict's unwillingness to seek help; covering up for the addict's behavior to employers, friends, and relatives; worrying about the addict's whereabouts and state of health; taking care of the addict's financial and legal problems, and so on. Living with an active addict can be living hell.

FAMILY DENIAL AND ENABLING:
WHEN HELPING HURTS

At some point in the addict's drug-use "career," family members begin to "buy into" the addict's own denial of the problem, forfeiting their own sense of reality. This is most likely to occur in family members who find (unconsciously) that focusing on the addict provides them with welcomed relief and distraction from their own problems, crises, and unhappiness. Why do families so often adopt denial? Members may harbor deep-seated guilt and fears that would inevitably be stimulated if they accepted the fact that their loved one is an addict: "I must have failed as a parent/spouse—I must have done something wrong"; "He/she must not really love or care about me"; or "There's no way out of this horrible problem; it's hopeless and incurable." Sometimes having a drug problem in the family causes profound feelings of shame: "What will our friends, relatives, and neighbors think? What would they say if they found out?" To admit that the drug problem exists, then, may mean having to experience this shame, and so the reality is blocked from consciousness.

For those who have lived their entire lifetimes blocking feelings from awareness, denial of a drug problem in the family may be an automatic and natural response: "If I ignore the problem, it will go away." This may actually work for a while in blocking feelings, but with a drug abuser in the family outside evidence of the problem will undoubtedly keep mounting, causing more and more anxiety to the family member trying to deny the problem. The discrepancy mounts between what he or she wants to believe and the tangible evidence of lost jobs, missing money, or arrests.

In response to this discrepancy many families begin trying to keep the crisis from occurring—at any cost. They want to keep the addict from losing the next job or keep the jewelry from disappearing in order better to maintain their own denial and avoid facing the problem and their feelings about it. This "damage control" behavior is sometimes carried to extremes, even by previously rational and otherwise "sane" people, as illustrated in the following case example.

When Mr. and Mrs. Lane came in for their first appointment, they described problems with their 15-year-old son, Tom, a cocaine addict. Over the course of the past year Tom had sold family antiques and jewelry, stolen from his parents, forged checks on their account, and damaged the family home extensively during wild "trashing" parties when he was left home alone. While they were on a recent vacation, he had made an unsuccessful suicide attempt (probably due to depression secondary to his chronic cocaine use) by taking an overdose of tranquilizers mixed with alcohol. During this year Mr. and Mrs. Lane had gradually but steadily dropped most of their leisure activities and interests in order to stand watch over Tom. At this point they had entirely given up their own social and private lives as a couple in order to take turns policing their son. These two bright and previously well-functioning people were living a miserable existence, heartbroken and terrified by their son's drug problem. They had become trapped in the "sick system" of an active addict: wanting to help, trying their best to do the "right thing" out of love and concern, and finding themselves not only unable to make things better but actually making things worse in the process. They had unwittingly become part of the problem as their lives more and more revolved around Tom—servicing his needs, cleaning up his "mess," and being obsessed with solving his problems rather than caring at all for themselves.

Sometimes family members' exaggerated focus on the addict is due in part to a lack of opportunity for objective feedback and "reality testing" about the situation. They are caught up in doing "what any loving mother/father/ spouse would do" when someone in the family has a problem. Much of this "enabling" behavior is an extension, albeit an exaggerated self-defeating one, of normal, socially encouraged caring/protective behavior toward loved ones. This is precisely what can make enabling so difficult to deal with— there are both moral and emotional imperatives that justify, rationalize, and drive this type of self-sacrificing behavior. Without informed feedback and education about addictive disease, family members usually assume almost total responsibility for the addict's problem and its resolution. Their self-esteem is eroded over time, both by this nagging sense of failure and by verbal or physical abuse from the addict, who is often masterful at aggravating feelings of guilt and assigning blame to others. Family members also find their own dispositions changing as they resort to nagging, pleading, and manipulating in their desperate but futile attempts to control the addict. Many end up despising their own behavior, further exacerbating feelings of guilt and shame.

As the above case example illustrates, when denying the problem is no longer enough to keep anxiety tolerable, family members may organize their lives around trying to control and manage the addict's behavior and problems. When family members or significant others (including therapists and other health professionals) behave, for whatever reason, in ways that directly or indirectly support, perpetuate, or facilitate the addict's drug use or drug-related behavior, it is called "enabling." Addictions cannot flourish in a vacuum. Family members who consciously or unconsciously collude with the addict in refusing to confront or even acknowledge the problem only serve to further the addiction. Once family members and others stop playing the enabler role, the addict is in trouble, since he or she requires a great deal of assistance in maintaining a distorted reality and in constantly arranging the environment to service addictive needs. Enabling includes a variety of different behavior patterns:

(1) *Minimizing*—rationalizing, ignoring, minimizing, or otherwise "explaining away" the addict's problem and its consequences: "It's not so bad; lots of people use drugs nowadays." "He's a troubled

person. He's had a tough life and needs a chance to work out his problems before he can stop using drugs."

(2) *Controlling* — attempting to manipulate or control the addict's drug supply and/or drug use; making bargains with the addict to be "good"; bribing the addict to stop using drugs; giving the addict ultimatums; making idle threats, etc.

(3) *Shielding* — protecting the addict from negative consequences of the addiction; making excuses, covering up, rescuing the addict from trouble, etc.

(4) *Taking over responsibilities* — paying bills, performing household tasks, etc.

(5) *Colluding* — helping the addict obtain drugs; giving the addict drugs.

Sometimes one family member hides the drug user's behavior from another (one parent hides it from the other, or a sibling hides it from the parents, for example). The person who colludes with the addict often rationalizes this behavior by assuming that if others were to find out about the drug use they would be too upset ("If Mom found out, she'd commit suicide") or respond too harshly and unreasonably toward the addict ("If Dad found out, he'd break your neck"). Sometimes keeping this "secret" produces secondary gains: It creates a special bond between the confidant and the addict.

What's Wrong With Enabling?

There is certainly nothing wrong with wanting to help a family member or friend in trouble, or even with "bending over backwards" and being somewhat self-sacrificing to help a loved one. It can be legitimately argued that in today's self-oriented society too few people are willing to sacrifice for others and help them with difficult problems. Helping behavior is commendable and should be encouraged.

However, sometimes helping hurts: when it is taken to an extreme and pursued compulsively in ways that make problems worse rather than better; when it impairs the functioning of the "helper"; and when it perpetuates the dependency and irresponsibility of the addict. People who persist in trying to help in ways that have not only proved to be futile, but are also negatively affecting both the addict and the helper are engaged in a pathological and potentially devastating process.

Family members of addicts are often embroiled in a desperate struggle trying to "save" their loved one from permanent damage or destruction. Deciding when to "help" and when to pull back and let the addict "fall on his/her face" can be an excruciatingly painful decision for parents and spouses, who often feel like they are in a "Catch-22" situation. If they continue trying to "help" the addict in their usual ways, he/she is spared some potentially horrendous consequences but never feels the "sting" of the addiction badly enough to be motivated to seek help and so continues to use drugs. On the other hand, if they stop enabling, the addict is likely to go further downhill into the depths of desperation and despair and be extremely angry and accusatory, but may eventually acquire the motivation to face his/her addiction.

Neither option is a perfect solution. Both involve sacrifices and potential dangers. Both involve uncertainty, since there is no way to predict or guarantee the outcome. When family members stop enabling, some addicts "turn around" very quickly and enter treatment without causing themselves a great deal of additional suffering. On the other hand, some get a lot worse and stay that way for a long time; some come close to dying; some actually die. It's no wonder that family members often feel that they are being "held hostage" by their loved one's addiction. They usually require a great deal of support, encouragement, and constructive guidance in order to face the problem squarely. The following case examples serve to further illustrate some of these points.

Addicted to cocaine for the past six years and currently unemployed Suzanne, a 37-year-old television production assistant, was arrested for passing bad checks, which she had done to get money for cocaine. Her father, an attorney residing in a different part of the country, flew in on the next plane and through local political connections retained an influential lawyer who managed to have all charges against Suzanne dropped. This was not the first time that Suzanne's father had bailed her out of trouble for drug-related behavior. She previously had been arrested for driving his car while intoxicated and for shoplifting in a department store. Both times her father "smoothed things over" to spare Suzanne (and probably himself as well) embarrassment and further hassles. For the past six years, he had been paying Suzanne's rent and her credit card bills, which typically amounted to more than $2,000 per month.

Suzanne's father stuck rigidly to the hope that somehow she would "see the light" and stop using drugs if he could just keep her life free of unnecessary problems and traumas. After all, he said, her mother had died when she was only nine years old and the deep emotional scars of that trauma would be with her for the rest of her life. In addition, he felt guilty about not being available enough to Suzanne after her mother died—he had immersed himself compulsively in his professional career and became a full-blown workaholic as a way to escape from his own sadness and pain.

After the most recent incident, Suzanne's drug use escalated dramatically. Previously restricting her use of cocaine to snorting only, she had now switched to freebasing after being introduced to it by a new boyfriend (himself an addict and drug dealer). Her drinking also escalated as the rebound depressions from high-dose cocaine use intensified. While intoxicated on cocaine and alcohol she and her boyfriend got into a violent argument. He beat her severely and left her alone in the apartment with a broken nose and two broken ribs, taking most of her expensive jewelry.

When Suzanne's father came to see her in the hospital emergency room, he was struck by the realization that he had actually helped Suzanne get to this miserable point in her life. He was determined to change the situation. He told her that, as sorry as he was to see her injured and in pain, he was no longer willing to let things just continue. He told Suzanne that unless she entered a drug treatment program upon being discharged from the hospital, he would no longer pay her rent or give her any money whatsoever. He felt a bit shaky inside saying this to her and knew he would need outside support and professional help in order to follow through on his good intentions.

Was it wrong of Suzanne's father to continuously bail her out of trouble and pay her basic living expenses? Would she have sought help and stopped using drugs sooner if he had not been enabling her? There is no way to know for sure. Suzanne's father did what most caring fathers would do in this same predicament. He tried to keep his daughter from suffering unpleasant and potentially life-damaging consequences of addictive behavior, hoping that she would somehow heed the warning signals and come to her senses before things got a lot worse. After all, he thought, wasn't the sheer anxiety and fear of possibly going to jail or having a criminal record enough to motivate her to seek help? Evidently not. Actually, Suzanne didn't experience any of these unpleasant feelings and didn't believe that the consequences would ever be imposed upon her anyway. She was "numbed out" by drugs and felt invulnerable because of her father's ability to shield her from trouble, as revealed in the following statement she made in a group session:

My father always seemed totally "freaked out" when I got in trouble. He was nervous, restless, and angry. He ran around like a nut, trying to clean up my mess. I knew I didn't have to deal with any of it — I could just sit back, ignore the whole thing, and let him take care of it. I'd say to myself: He's a master at solving difficult problems — that's what he does for a living—he solves other people's problems. So why not mine? And sure enough, he would always come through for me. I had no anxiety, no fears about the problems—he had enough for both of us. I didn't have to do or feel anything. He took care of everything and did a great job of it. What's more, I was totally distracted by drugs. I remember sitting in the courtroom 2,000 miles from home thinking about how I was going to get high as soon as I got out of there—meanwhile my Dad was shuffling papers, talking to the judge, trying to pull all the strings to get me out of the mess—and there I was daydreaming about drugs, not doing a damn thing to help myself. I felt that nothing bad could ever really happen to me. I had someone who made sure of that.

Suzanne's statement highlights the major problem with enabling behavior: It creates and fosters a self-defeating illusion. It allows addicts to feel invulnerable, omnipotent, unique, and powerful—as if the laws that govern the universe apply to everyone but them. Obviously, this is dangerous thinking. It allows addicts to continue or even escalate their destructive behavior, believing that they will suffer no consequences.

Deciding when to set limits on the addict and focus instead on one's own needs can be very difficult for family members, as shown in the case of Helen, a drug abuse counselor in a local treatment center, who despite her professional knowledge severely enabled the cocaine addiction of her husband, Ken. Hoping that they wouldn't have to default on their home mortgage, she escorted Ken to work everyday to insure that he got there, made excuses for his absenteeism when he refused to get out of bed, borrowed money from her parents, and "juggled" the family finances. With professional help, she decided that the only way she could change the situation was to help herself. If it ended up helping Ken at the same time, that would be great, but she had to focus on herself first. She entered our family counseling program and simultaneously joined a support group (Coc-Anon). She closed her joint bank with Ken, established a separate account of her own, notified Ken's parents and brothers about the problem, and refused to allow him back into their house until he got straight and got help.

Ken reacted with outrage at being thrown out of his own home and "abandoned" by his wife. He entered the house when Helen was at work, stole several pieces of her jewelry and took the family car. Helen subsequently changed the locks and notified Ken that the next time he entered the house or took anything from her, she would report him to the police and seek a restraining order from the court. Ken spent the next two months living in "crack houses." He would call Helen every week or so and plead with her to let him come back home, but she was unyielding until he finally entered a treatment program.

Sometimes, family members deny that their behavior is enabling the patient's drug use to continue. They selectively focus on their efforts to provide the addict with the "bare necessities" of living — food, shelter, clothing — saying, "How can anyone expect him/her to have any hope and optimism for the future or even try to get a job if he has no place to live, no food to eat, and no decent clothing to wear? Isn't that helping rather than hurting?"

The case of Donna, a 27-year-old unemployed graphic artist, illustrates this point. Donna's parents, suspecting that she had a drug problem, were careful not to give her cash that could be used to buy drugs, but instead assumed certain other expenses for her, including rent, food, and credit card bills that they paid directly. Donna's parents had difficulty realizing that, even though they were not giving her money explicitly for cocaine, they were nonetheless enabling her drug use by paying for other expenses. The money she didn't have to pay for these other expenses directly subsidized her drug use. Enabling, as the term implies, allows the addict to continue using drugs, however directly or indirectly the case may be. By making drug use easier, shielding the addict from its consequences and colluding with the problem, family members end up adding fuel to the fire.

CO-DEPENDENCY

It may be quite normal for concerned family members to engage temporarily in some form of enabling behavior in response to a loved one's addiction — at least until the "enabler" sees what's really going on (i.e., that helping is actually hurting) and before the situation "backfires" out of control. But family members who chronically continue this destructive course of action have a more serious and more permanent problem called "co-dependency." Someone who suffers from co-dependency characteristically gets compulsively and obsessively involved in the problems of the addict (or others), to the point where this behavior seriously and chronically damages the quality of his/her life. The primary addict is addicted to drugs while the co-addict or co-dependent is addicted to the addict's problems.

The major features of co-dependency include the following:

(1) Co-dependency is increasingly understood as an addiction of its own, characterized by the same symptoms:

 (a) a loss of control over the behavior;

 (b) compulsivity;

 (c) continuation of the behavior despite adverse consequences;

 (d) denial that the problem exists. In addition, the co-dependent becomes progressively tolerant of the addict's increasingly aberrant and self-destructive behavior.

(2) The developmental course or progression of the co-dependency problem parallels that of the drug addiction problem.

(3) Among those at highest risk for developing co-dependency problems are individuals who are themselves stressed or unhappy due to their own life crises/problems or psychiatric illness, and/or those who characteristically employ exaggerated maladaptive defenses (especially denial) in their attempts to cope with serious problems.

(4) Co-dependency is more likely to occur in families where significant interpersonal problems exist. For example, parents who have troubled marriages are more likely to compulsively focus on their son's or daughter's addiction, partly because it diverts attention from their own problem.

(5) Co-dependency is encouraged to some extent by our cultural norms of what "nice, caring people" do. A wife who sticks by her cocaine-addicted spouse, picks up the pieces, and covers up for him while at the same time trying to hold the family together financially and emotionally is often given a lot of credit by friends and relatives, even though her enabling behavior makes the situation even worse. The co-dependent's illusion of being dedicated, self-sacrificing, and limitlessly caring may help bolster sagging self-esteem.

IMPACT OF COCAINE ADDICTION VS. ALCOHOLISM

Most of the existing self-help and professional literature on families and chemical dependency focuses almost entirely on alcoholism. Very little has been written about the special problems of families affected by cocaine addiction. Although cocaine and alcohol addictions share many similarities, there are noteworthy differences between the two drugs (as discussed in Chapter 5), which create different problems for the respective families of cocaine addicts and alcoholics. Most of these differences stem from the fact that the progression from an individual's first use of cocaine to full-blown cocaine addiction is usually much more rapid than that from an individual's first drink to full-blown alcoholism. A freebase or crack smoker, for example, can become addicted in a matter of weeks or months, and even cocaine snorters can get addicted within a couple of years. The alcoholic, on the other hand, may drink over a period of 10 to 15 years before showing clear-cut signs of addiction. Of course, for teens the progression to either addiction tends to occur much more rapidly.

In what ways is cocaine addiction different from alcoholism in affecting the family? First of all, there is often a striking, rapid change in the cocaine addict's behavior and personality. The sharp contrast, within a relatively short period of time, between the addict's behavior on vs. off the drug can reveal the presence of the addiction in an obvious, dramatic way. With alcohol, the family often goes through a prolonged period of asking themselves: "How much drinking is really too much?" and saying, "Well, yeah, he drinks a bit too much at times, but doesn't everyone?" With cocaine, the addict's disrupted functioning, extreme personality/mood changes, and overwhelming obsession with the drug tend to reveal the presence of the problem more readily. In addition, since relatives of the cocaine addict usually haven't lived with the problem for a long time, they have not gone through an extensive "adjustment" period where they have accommodated to the problem and lost perspective on how bizarre and abnormal the addict's behavior really is. Although cocaine-affected families are just as likely to engage in enabling behavior as alcoholic families, as the above examples illustrate, the co-dependent patterns and family roles may not yet be as solidly entrenched; perhaps, therefore, they are at least sometimes more easily reversed.

Denial occurs in the family of the cocaine addict, to be sure. But like the enabling, it usually has not had as much time to become woven into the family fabric and may, therefore, be somewhat easier to break with outside help. The family member of a cocaine addict, while drawn into the family disease of addiction and acting in the characteristic ways of the co-dependent, is nevertheless likely to maintain some level of self-perception. It's not unusual for an enabling spouse, or parent to say something like, "This is crazy! I know I shouldn't be acting this way. I'm doing things I don't even want to do, but I don't seem to be able to stop!"

A second difference stems from the fact that cocaine is illegal and, therefore, may be less tolerated by family members than alcohol. Most parents and spouses of cocaine users are likely to confront a cocaine problem sooner than they would a developing alcohol problem. Cocaine poses a more obvious, identifiable threat to the user's career and holds the possibility of arrest and incarceration, whereas alcohol is socially accepted and even promoted. Using illegal drugs is generally considered to be more devious and more dangerous than drinking alcohol so that family members often feel more justified in demanding that their loved one stop using the drug immediately.

A third difference is that during initial involvement with cocaine its use generally does not disrupt a person's functioning as noticeably as that of alcohol. There is no telltale breath odor from using cocaine, no stumbling gait, slurred speech, or general lack of coordination. In addition, someone high on cocaine is likely to be talkative and congenial, not boisterous and belligerent. The beginning cocaine user, then, is often able to hide his/her use from the family altogether until a crisis of some sort reveals it. In these cases, discovery of the cocaine use may come as a total surprise to the family — especially when the cocaine user is a teenager. There are many cases where a wife has had no knowledge whatsoever of her husband's cocaine use until an arrest or medical emergency occurs. What this means for treatment is simply that family members' "denial" may reflect a genuine lack of awareness of the problem. Clinicians should be aware of this possibility.

WHICH FAMILY MEMBERS SHOULD BE INVOLVED?

Involving the family in the addict's treatment is often essential to achieving success. However, it may not always be possible to get the family involved. Some adult patients are far removed from their families geographically and/or emotionally and some have no mate and no living parents. Others strongly resist involving their families at first or at all. Still other patients are receptive to the idea of involving their family, but the family refuses to be involved: They prefer to "wash their hands" of the whole situation, feel that they've been taken enough advantage of by the addict, don't feel optimistic that anything will help the addict, don't have time to be involved because of work or career responsibilities, or are fearful and anxious that they will be blamed by the addict and the program staff for the problem.

Suggestions for handling some of these situations will be discussed below, but first let's address the question of which family members (or significant others) should be actively encouraged to participate in the patient's treatment. The following are some general guidelines, although exceptions often exist:

(1) Anyone who lives in the same household with the addict.

(2) Anyone who provides financial assistance, directly or indirectly, to the addict.

(3) Anyone who is significantly involved in managing the addict's finances or making major life decisions with/for the addict.

(4) Any intimately involved spouse or mate.

(5) Anyone who is seriously enabling the addict (including an employer).

(6) Anyone who is genuinely concerned about the addict and wants to be involved (e.g., friends, employers, neighbors).

Especially with adolescent patients, both parents should be urged to participate in treatment, even if they are separated or divorced. With teenage addicts, there is a high likelihood of one parent being played off against the other by the addict or of one disgruntled parent blaming the other for the problem in a way that sabotages treatment, unless both are involved in the process.

Are there instances where family members need not or distinctly should not be involved in the addict's treatment? Yes. Very young siblings or children of the addict need not be involved, depending upon to what extent their lives have been affected by the addict's behavior and whether they are emotionally and intellectually capable of dealing with the issue. Also, it is unnecessary and sometimes downright inadvisable to involve the family in certain cases — for example, when parents are elderly, sick, and neither contributing to nor suffering from the addict's problems, or when family members are destructively negative toward the addict and blatantly refuse to even consider changing their attitude or behavior. Some family members really do despise their addict relative and consistently do serious harm rather than good whenever they have any contact with him/her. In such cases, it is best to help the patient accept the reality of these destructive relationships and to effectively separate from them rather than unrealistically seek greater closeness. In some cases, family members are themselves so psychiatrically disturbed that they are incapable of providing any help.

HOW TO GET THE FAMILY INVOLVED

Some family members are highly resistant when asked to participate in the addict's treatment. They may feel hopeless and guilty; many are extraordinarily sensitive to feeling blamed. Common responses are: "Why do you want me to be involved? It's his/her problem, not mine," or, "I've done everything I can for him/her already; I don't think there's anything left for me to do."

Others are receptive and even enthusiastic about being involved. Despite feeling distraught and confused, they want very much to help and welcome an opportunity to receive advice and support in dealing with their relative's problem. Some seek help for themselves even though the addict has not yet entered or even accepted the need for treatment. They are usually motivated by a combination of wanting relief from their own suffering and a desire to try anything that might increase the chances that the addict will finally seek help.

The receptivity and willingness of family members to participate in the addict's treatment can be affected by exactly how the issue is presented to them. They are far more likely to accept an offer to obtain education and advice about the best ways to handle addiction problems in the family than an offer to receive therapy and counseling for their own "co-dependency" problems and inappropriate behavior toward the addict. The first step is to have a meeting with immediate family members to assess their individual and family situations and to determine their willingness and appropriateness for involvement in the program. Family members should not simply be thrown into a group without first being properly assessed.

FAMILY ASSESSMENT

The goals of the first meeting with family members are to:

(1) determine exactly what they do or don't know about the patient's addiction problem and obtain any additional information that either corroborates or refutes the patient's reported history;

(2) assess and explore how each family member and the entire family system have been affected by the addict's problem;

(3) provide an opportunity for them to ventilate some of their anger, frustration, and other negative feelings;

(4) assess the extent of their enabling behavior and co-dependency problems, including the full spectrum of personal consequences they have suffered as a result of the patient's addiction; and

(5) describe a basic strategy or treatment plan for addressing these problems, including a preliminary explanation of enabling behavior and the value of being part of a family support group.

The initial assessment covers a wide range of topics, as shown in the Family Questionnaire (Appendix H), a self-administered intake form that is completed in the waiting room by each family member just prior to the initial interview. Topics covered in the form include:

(1) their knowledge about the patient's past and present drug use and treatment;

(2) their current belief about the severity and causes of the addict's problem;

(3) how they have attempted so far to help the addict, as assessed in a lengthy checklist of possible enabling behaviors;

(4) how their own mood, mental state, physical health, social life, sex life, relationships, and finances have been affected by the addict's problems, as assessed in an extensive checklist of possible consequences;

(5) their own history of past and present drug/alcohol use, psychological problems, and any treatment for such problems; and

(6) their degree of optimism or pessimism about the addict's chances for recovery and how they might respond if the addict relapses.

Some of the key issues raised in the assessment interview are outlined below:

(1) How has your relative's addiction affected you?
   (a) Emotionally. (Mood swings, irritability, withdrawing from friends and activities, depression, loss of sex drive, displacing anger onto others, etc.)
   (b) Physically. (Stress-related illnesses, low energy, loss of appetite or compulsive eating, loss of interest in physical appearance, etc.)
   (c) Financially. (Belongings sold by the addict, legal fees or debts paid for the addict, depletion of bank accounts, sale of assets, income loss due to crisis-ridden existence, etc.)
   (d) Socially. (Becoming isolated from friends and family, shift of attention from own interests and hobbies to addict's behavior and crises, etc.)

(2) What strategies for coping have you tried, and what effect have these attempts had on you? (Blocking it out, ignoring it, blaming, manipulating, using guilt, blowing up, vigilance and detective work, etc.)

(3) How has your family restructured itself in attempting to deal with the addict and a chronic sense of crisis? (Children taking over some of the parents' roles, wife taking over husband's role or vice versa, kids asking less attention because they see parents are preoccupied, members becoming more isolated from each other or more united, etc.)

(4) Have you ever found yourself feeling like you should cover up for the addict, bail him/her out of trouble, pay bills, etc.?

(5) What is your current attitude toward the addict and his/her problem? (Fed up, don't feel can be a support, glad he/she is getting help, want to get behind him/her and learn as much as possible, "too little too late," in shock and don't know yet, etc.)

(6) What if the addict relapses or fails to recover? (Will you "give up" on him/her, will you be very angry, will you throw him out of the house, will you feel hopeless, etc.)

(7) What do you expect from treatment — for yourself and for your addicted relative? (It will cure him/her; nothing, it probably won't

help very much, etc.) (Unrealistic expectations will be revealed. This is a good time for education about the recovery process — that there may be relapses, that it may be difficult, that progress may be slow and will take time, etc.)

TREATMENT PROGRAM

Family members who enter our outpatient treatment program participate in an eight-week education group for spouses and parents (no primary patients are present) and simultaneously participate in a multiple family group consisting of several patients and their respective family members together. After completing the eight-week program family members have the option of continuing in an open-ended group, with separate groups for spouses and parents, who at this stage usually have different concerns, i.e., parenting issues vs. marital and sexual issues.

The eight-week education group has a structured rotating "syllabus" designed to teach family members about addictive disease, the medical and pharmacological aspects of addictive drugs, and the basic principles of recovery, relapse, co-dependency, and enabling. A combination of lectures, films, slides, readings, homework assignments, and topic-oriented discussions is used. The multiple family group is less structured and more experiential. It provides an opportunity to expose and address enabling behaviors, family conflicts, and communication problems. Family members and addicts are free to bring up any issue for discussion, although the group leaders often guide and focus the discussions in order to maximize understanding of certain key issues (e.g., enabling behavior, relapse, negative feelings, sabotage) as they arise spontaneously in the group. Some group sessions begin with a stated topic, psychodrama, or family "sculpting" techniques.

Treatment Goals

Just as the development of co-dependency parallels that of primary addiction, so do the major goals and stages of family treatment/recovery, as outlined below:

(1) *Establish initial abstinence from enabling.* The first and foremost treatment goal is for family members to achieve initial abstinence from all enabling behaviors. In most cases, this is not accomplished immediately, but in gradual steps as family members ventilate negative feelings (anger, hurt, guilt, shame, resentment, etc.), gain an understanding of enabling, identify their own enabling behaviors, and ultimately feel confident that eliminating these behaviors will help both the addict and themselves. Although addicts must immediately stop using drugs when they enter a treatment program,

co-dependents usually require preliminary education and supportive counseling before they can even consider "pulling back" from their enabling behavior. Usually, when family members first come to treatment, while they already realize that the addict has a problem, they either have not yet realized or have difficulty admitting that they too have a problem—that they are an integral part of a system that keeps the addiction going.

(2) *Provide basic education about addictive disease as both an individual and family problem.* Part of the effort to help family members achieve initial abstinence from enabling is to provide basic education about the family dynamics of addictive disease. Here it is best to focus primarily on how the family members respond to the addict's problem and how they end up adjusting their own behavior to it in ways that unwittingly perpetuate the problem. It is counterproductive to emphasize how the "sick" and maladaptive interaction in the family caused the problem in the first place, for even if it is partly true, it only heightens the family's resistance. It is essential to keep the focus on present rather than past behavior and to avoid unnecessarily stimulating further guilt. A relevant slogan from Al-Anon reminds family members of the "three C's": You didn't *cause* your loved one's addiction, you can't *control* it, and you can't *cure* it. Family members are encouraged to "detach with love," that is, to stop participating in the addict's problem and remove themselves from this destructive situation out of love and concern for the addict and for themselves—not out of anger, hatred, and revenge.

Family members are usually very interested in learning about the medical and psychological consequences of cocaine use, but are at first prone to using this information in counterproductive ways. For example, some use it to justify their anger at the addict for being so "self-destructive" and for "stupidly" ignoring the well-documented harmful consequences of chronic cocaine use. Until family members come to accept the disease model of addiction and their inability (powerlessness) to control the addict's behavior, they often remain stuck in the vicious cycle of enabling and co-dependency. It's often easier to think of a loved one as temporarily "bad" rather than permanently "sick."

To overcome these tendencies, it helps to explain the biological aspects of addictive disease in general and cocaine addiction in particular, especially the effects of cocaine on brain function, which impair the addict's reasoning abilities and create overwhelming cravings and urges for the drug that are physical, not just psychological. Family members are often able to be more empathic toward the addict and to let go of overly negative and unhelpful feelings that block their understanding of the problem when they realize that much of the addict's destructive behavior is characteristic of the active disease and not necessarily characteristic of the diseased person. However, it is just as important to emphasize that addicts are nonetheless responsible for their behavior, even though they are not responsible for having the disease that distorts their behavior when active. Family members who have suffered greatly as a result of the addict's behavior are often highly resistant to accepting the disease model. They feel that to do so would just give the addict an excuse (pardon) for past behavior and a justification for returning to drugs in the future. As with addicts themselves, helping family members to go beyond an intellectual understanding of addiction to achieve a deeper emotional acceptance of the problem is essential to lasting success.

(3) *Prevent relapse to enabling.* Once initial abstinence from enabling behavior is achieved, the next goal is to prevent "relapse": the tendency or "pull" for family members to return to enabling and other co-dependent behaviors, especially if the addict relapses to drugs, but also when the addict continues to stay drug-free. Family members must be helped to see the multiple functions served by their enabling behavior, including their "vested interest" in perpetuating their loved one's addiction, which they consciously detest, but which serves nonetheless to deflect attention away from personal and family problems and to maintain the "status quo."

Similar to the relapse process in primary addiction, there are relapse risk factors and warning signs of co-dependency that must be addressed. These include:

(1) negative mood states, especially feelings of depression resulting from the "paradoxical loss" that occurs when the whirlwind involvement in activities surrounding the addict's problems abruptly ceases (some family members are left with no substitute activities to keep them preoccupied and distracted from their own problems and empty existence);

(2) feeling that the recovering addict is basically "cured" and refusing to face the possibility that he/she might ever relapse;

(3) colluding with the addict in believing that cocaine but not alcohol is a threat to his/her recovery—and possibly offering the addict "benign" drinks such as wine or beer at dinners and parties;

(4) giving the recovering addict gifts or "rewards" for being abstinent, such as money or jewelry, that supply renewed access to cocaine;

(5) acting out negative feelings toward the recovering addict, such as anger about previous hurtful acts and resentment or jealousy about all the help and attention he/she is now receiving while the family member feels like the major victim of the addict's problems;

(6) missing or coming late to family sessions and/or planning to drop out of the program prematurely;

(7) sabotaging the recovering addict's treatment by deciding not to

continue paying for it (although the family can reasonably afford it) or, in cases where the addict is employed in a family business, refusing to arrange the addict's working hours to allow him/her to participate in treatment;

(8) protecting the recovering addict from stress and upset out of fear that he/she will return to drugs and in the process fostering the addict's dependency and making him/her feel helpless and infantilized.

(4) *Address personal and family problems.* After the above goals have been achieved and the family situation has "settled down," there is an opportunity for family members to address some of their own personal and emotional problems, especially those that continue to diminish the quality of their lives and make them prime targets for co-dependency. For example, many have themselves grown up in families with addiction problems (involving drugs, food, sex, gambling, etc.), psychiatric problems, or other types of family dysfunction that promote co-dependent behavior and distort one's personality. Even in the absence of such family histories, they may suffer from problems of identity/role confusion, life crises, psychological distortions, maladaptive coping strategies, and sexual difficulties.

Sometimes there are serious marital problems to be addressed, while among the parents of adult addicts it is not unusual to find that one or both parents are struggling with life crises and problems stemming from current or anticipated retirement, chronic and debilitating illness, or the "empty nest" syndrome. Wives of addicts are often suffering from chronically low self-esteem and other consequences of habitually giving low priority to their own needs. Special groups for the wives and girlfriends of addicts, led by female therapists, provide a very effective and "safe" place for these women to share, ventilate, and receive constructive feedback and support about their self-defeating behavior and how to change it. Separate groups for the parents of addicts serve a similar function in providing an opportunity for role modeling, peer support, and professional guidance, but with the focus primarily on parenting, marital, and life-crisis issues. Participation in these spouse or parents groups is either supplemented or replaced, where indicated, with individual, couples, or family therapy sessions.

There is a continuing debate in the addiction treatment field about whether co-dependency is itself a permanent disease for which there is only recovery and no cure and whether it requires long-term treatment and/or participation in self-help programs such as Coc-Anon or Al-Anon. There is an even more fundamental disagreement about whether addicts' families of origin, without exception, always represent disturbed family systems that inevitably give rise to addiction problems.

Based on purely clinical rather than theoretical considerations, therapists should adopt whatever approach works. Many families who balk at having the disease model of co-dependency shoved down their throats still readily accept and make good use of concepts about enabling and co-dependency. Moreover, some families show very little enabling behavior and virtually no serious co-dependency problems. Especially with parents of adult addicts (particularly older adults, age 30 and over) it is unhelpful to focus on where their child-rearing practices or family dynamics may have gone wrong: this approach holds little possibility for benefit and much possibility for harm. As for family self-help programs, they are almost always useful, and participation should be actively encouraged. But families who do not attend these programs should not be written off as resistant, noncompliant, and hopeless. Making Coc-Anon or Al-Anon meetings available on the premises of the treatment program or clinic is one way to foster involvement.

Family Groups

The basic core of the family treatment program consists of two groups, one exclusively for family members and one for addicts and family members together, both of which run concurrently for eight consecutive weeks. The effectiveness of group treatment for family members stems from the unique benefits and opportunities it offers for peer support, as well as experiential and imitative learning, as outlined below:

(1) *Ventilation and reduced isolation.* By hearing others who have been through similar experiences, new members quickly feel less unique, less isolated, more accepting of their feelings, and less self-blaming.

(2) *Learning about the family disease of addiction.* By observing that their own behavioral and emotional responses to a loved one's addiction have been very similar to those of other families, members can be helped to see that addiction usually involves the entire family and that their responses to it are not "crazy" and unusual. Feelings of shame and stigmatization are reduced and a sense of relief often ensues.

(3) *Increased awareness of enabling behavior.* As others in the group discuss and expose their enabling behavior, newer members hear familiar patterns and become more willing to acknowledge their own enabling behavior. Members can begin to accept their own need to recover and to change their behavior.

(4) *Role modeling for limit-setting.* Families at a later stage of the program provide role models for becoming more assertive, setting limits, and ending enabling. Newer members can begin to learn more effective communication skills, regain self-respect, and receive positive feedback and support in approaching these difficult tasks.

(5) *Support for focusing on oneself.* Senior members also provide role models for placing the focus back on oneself. As these members speak with vitality about their own interests, careers, hobbies, social events, and so on, new members begin to see the hope of recovery and are helped to begin taking the focus off the addict.

(6) *Reinforcement of the idea of having a choice.* The overall effect of the group is to serve as a reminder to members that they do have choices as to how they are going to respond to the addictive illness: to stop enabling the addict and to accept their powerlessness over the addict's disease; to allow the addict to experience the consequences of his/her own drug use; to relinquish efforts to control the addict's recovery; and to focus on themselves and their own lives instead of someone else's.

(7) *Instillation of hope and optimism.* Ultimately, the living example of families at a further stage of recovery helps others to feel optimistic and hopeful about the possibility of having a better life—regardless of whether or not the addict gets well.

Help With Feelings

When family members come into treatment they are often overwhelmed by a complex of negative feelings that must be addressed in treatment.

FEAR

Family members harbor intense fears about the addict, about themselves, and about the family as a whole. They live in a tortured state, with an uncertain and unpredictable outcome. They fear that the addict will hurt or kill him/herself, hurt others in the family in a fit of rage, or send the family into financial ruin. They fear standing up to the addict and the prospect that stopping their enabling behavior will make things worse instead of better.

GUILT

It is often hard for family members to get in touch with their deep-seated feelings of guilt. They feel personally responsible for their loved one's addiction and believe that, if only they had done things differently, everything now would be fine. Many secretly wish that the addict would just die and put an end to the whole miserable situation—and they feel guilty for harboring these unacceptable wishes.

SHAME

The family often feels stigmatized and shamed by the addict. They are riddled with conflicting feelings of shame and loving concern. Shame exacerbates denial and fosters the pretense that everything's "just fine."

GRIEF

There is a profound sense of grief when parents of the addict feel that they lost the opportunity to have a "normal" son or daughter. Similarly, spouses of addicts feel that they have lost the opportunity to have a "normal" marriage. Grief also stems from seeing that the person they once knew and enjoyed being with is now very different and very unappealing — and perhaps will be forever.

ANGER

There is usually a great deal of anger toward the addict — feelings that he or she has shamed the family, that the family has been manipulated and abused, that family members have been forsaken for the "love" of cocaine. Especially when family members have not yet had the opportunity to understand addictive disease, they tend to see the addiction as self-inflicted rather than outside of the addict's control, and feel angry that he/she has "chosen" to do this to him/herself and the family.

If the above feelings are not identified and addressed in treatment, they can negatively influence both the addict's and the family's recovery. Bottled-up feelings create an atmosphere of tension in the home, impede communication, and prohibit expression of the compassion and caring that family members often have toward their loved one — robbing the addict of a valuable source of support in recovery. Furthermore, unexpressed feelings of hostility, resentment, and fear can be acted out by family members in a way that could sabotage the addict's treatment, as the following case example illustrates.

Brian, a 17-year-old cocaine addict, had been in the outpatient treatment program for a month. Attempts to involve his divorced parents in the program were unsuccessful. They either didn't return phone calls or separately made appointments for an initial interview but cancelled them at the last minute. Mrs. Thomas called without warning to say that she was withdrawing Brian from the program because she didn't think that he needed it any longer. Brian's therapist urged her to at least come in to discuss the matter in person before carrying out her decision. No attempt was made to talk her out of the decision on the telephone. She agreed to a meeting. When she arrived for the meeting later that week, she leveled a string of harsh and irrational criticisms about the treatment program, which the therapist did not attempt to suppress. During this tirade, the therapist listened attentively with an open, nondefensive posture that neither joined Mrs. T. in her disparaging of the program nor defended it. The therapist simply replied with a statement about how difficult it must be for her to realize that her son had a serious, though treatable, problem.

Mrs. Thomas immediately broke into tears, explaining how she felt not only worried about Brian, but caught between him and his stepfather, a no-nonsense sort of man who was strongly opposed to therapy and to spending any money on it. She felt that her new marriage was severely threatened by Brian's drug use. She had conflicting feelings of resentment and caring. She agreed to attend family groups and eventually her new husband entered the program as well, as did Brian's biological father, who attended a separate group and conjoint family therapy sessions with his son and former wife. It was the initial ventilation of Mrs. T.'s displaced anger that provided the turning point and allowed significant changes to take place.

Table 10.1 lists key points for the family to remember. These incorporate many of the issues discussed in this chapter.

TABLE 10.1
Points for the Family to Remember

1. You are not to blame for the addict's disease. You didn't cause it, you can't control it, and you can't cure it.
2. While you are not to blame for the disease's existence, you are responsible for your own behavior. You have the choice to refrain from enabling the addict's drug use and drug-related behavior.
3. Your relative's addiction is not a sign of family weakness or disgrace and can happen in any family, just like other diseases.
4. Don't nag, preach, moralize, threaten, or blame the addict for past and present mistakes. You only make yourself the target of the addict's anger and frustration, and do nothing to change his/her behavior.
5. Don't cover up, make excuses, or otherwise try to protect the addict from the natural consequences of his/her behavior. In doing so you become an accomplice (enabler) in perpetuating the addict's drug use and irresponsible behavior. Addicts are more likely to seek help when the pain of using drugs becomes worse to bear than the pain of not using.
6. Don't try to "play shrink" or make psychological excuses for the addict's behavior. The addiction should not be blamed on childhood traumas, job stress, or marital problems that must be resolved before the addict can stop using drugs. This just gives the addict further justification to continue using.
7. Don't search for, hide, or throw away the addict's drug supplies or paraphernalia. The addict will inevitably just get more. Trying to keep him or her away from drug-using friends won't work either.
8. Don't lay guilt trips on the addict in an attempt to get him/her to stop using. Saying things like "if you really loved me, you would stop doing this to yourself" only creates negative feelings that give the addict more excuses to use drugs. Guilt doesn't work.

(continued)

TABLE 10.1 (Continued)

9. Don't use idle threats as a means of manipulation. You can and should set limits, but first think them through carefully and then be fully prepared to follow through. If you don't mean what you say, don't say it. The addict only learns that you are full of "hot air" and will further discount you.

10. Don't accept the addict's hollow promises to be "good" or accept a few days off drugs, a single visit to a doctor, or a telephone call to a program with no follow-through as evidence that the addict is serious about getting help. Stick with what the addict does, not what he/she says.

11. Don't allow the addict to exploit you monetarily or otherwise. Protect yourself. Maintain your dignity and self-respect.

12. Don't ignore or overlook lying and other forms of deceitful and manipulative behavior. Don't collude with the addict in keeping secrets about drug use from the therapist or program. To do so only assists the addict in evasion of responsibility for his/her behavior and perpetuates the problem.

13. Don't be jealous and resentful of the addict's newfound recovering friends and support system, even if his/her involvement with them reduces your time together. This is a vital and indispensable part of his/her recovery. Join your own support group, make new friends, develop new leisure activities.

14. Don't delude yourself into thinking that the addict is "cured" and will never use drugs again, no matter how good he/she is doing right now. Imagine and think through a relapse scenario and how you would handle it.

15. Don't be diverted from focusing on yourself. Use the support system and resources available to you to foster your recovery from co-dependency.

16. Don't try to protect the recovering person from normal family problems.

17. Don't try to control the addict's recovery by checking up on appointments, calling sponsors, nagging about not going to meetings, etc. Don't ask for reports about the content of his/her counseling sessions.

18. Don't overreact to possible signs of relapse in the addict. Bring them up calmly and directly, without accusation.

19. Don't act-out feelings of being left behind by the addict. After putting up with all the crises of addiction, you may feel lonely and less needed when he/she enters treatment.

20. Don't expect the recovering person to be cheerful all the time now and don't overreact to his/her bad moods with fears about relapse. Allow him/her the latitude to be irritable, anxious, and unhappy, etc., without having it create a crisis.

21. Don't expect the addict's cessation of drug use to solve all family problems. Other problems—some of which were ignored, set aside, or avoided while the whole family focused on the active addict—are likely to surface and become evident.

22. Don't ignore your own relapse warning signs. Your enabling behavior and co-dependency problems are likely to show up again at some point, but you can "short-circuit" them if you know what to look for.

CHAPTER 11

Treating Special Populations

THIS FINAL CHAPTER deals with treating cocaine addiction in special populations: adolescents, women, health-care professionals, and athletes.

ADOLESCENTS

An increasing number of adolescents try cocaine, begin using it occasionally, and get addicted to it. It is more easily available to teenagers than ever before and now, with the advent of crack, there is an even greater likelihood that occasional use will lead to addiction.

Unfortunately, using cocaine has become one of the ways that today's teenagers imitate adults in their persistent quest to be grown-up. Cocaine is appealing to teens partly because it has a high-status trendy image, but it's more than that—cocaine temporarily supplies many of the feelings that are highly valued and desired by adolescents. Cocaine instantly makes the user feel more talkative, outgoing, confident, assertive, sociable, and adventurous. Shyness, awkwardness, hesitation, and sexual anxiety may magically disappear, at least in the early stage of use.

The importance adolescents place on "letting loose" makes a drug that reduces inhibitions and creates a "party" mood especially appealing to young people. Cocaine is the ultimate escape from negative mood states: Almost instantly upon using the drug, fear, frustration, depression, and feelings of loneliness seem to evaporate. Because adolescents are often malignantly attracted to high-risk activities, using a drug that is associated with certain well-known and well-publicized dangers may only add to cocaine's magnetic appeal.

Treatment Considerations

While the treatment techniques outlined in previous chapters are generally applicable to adolescents with minor adjustments, several issues deserve special consideration.

REASONS FOR ENTERING TREATMENT

Not unlike their adult counterparts, most teenage cocaine addicts come to treatment under severe pressure from others, in their case usually parents or school officials. Their motivation to enter a program may have more to do with a desire to regain certain privileges (e.g., use of the family car, later curfews) or to avoid the imposition of further consequences (e.g., suspension from school, being thrown out of their parents' home) than with a genuine desire for professional help. The clinician must be prepared to encounter a thick wall of resistance from a cocaine-addicted teenager, at least initially. In extreme cases, it may take two or three preliminary sessions before the adolescent is willing to conduct a conversation with the therapist and supply something more than one-word answers, let alone share any meaningful information about his/her drug use and other personal matters.

The clinician must be prepared to "start where the patient is" and to accept very small signs of progress in order to engage the adolescent cocaine addict into treatment. Power struggles must be avoided. If the adolescent's main reason for coming to treatment is to produce a few drug-free urines just to placate parents or school officials, the clinician can avoid strongly challenging this intention by "joining" with the patient. It is possible simultaneously to express deep concern about the potential consequences of continued drug use and empathy for the adolescent's distress about parents and other adults watching his/her every move. The trick is to somehow redefine achieving abstinence as a move toward independence rather than submission to the wishes of authority figures. Teenagers must be helped to see how abstinence can remove obstacles between them and what they want rather than be seen as a sign of defeat.

INPATIENT VS. OUTPATIENT TREATMENT

Most adolescent cocaine addicts do not require residential care and can be treated effectively in an intensive outpatient program. Usually, adolescents are especially fearful of residential programs because of the stigma they associate with having to be "put away" for a serious drug problem and because they do not want to be separated from their friends. Such fear often provides the motivation for an adolescent to make better use of outpatient treatment. However, some adolescents will need an inpatient setting from the very outset because of medical complications and/or severe psychosocial dysfunction. Others who fail to show sufficient progress in the early phase of outpatient treatment may also need inpatient care. This does not mean that a relapse during outpatient treatment is in itself sufficient reason to insist that the adolescent enter a hospital. Such decisions must be based on an overall assessment of the patient's progress, attitude, and current level of psychosocial functioning.

FAMILY INVOLVEMENT

Involving the family in the treatment of the adolescent is essential because usually parents, no matter how temporarily estranged, continue to have enormous influence on the adolescent's life. Parents often control the adolescent's access to treatment in very pragmatic ways, such as providing money and/or transportation. A sibling who uses drugs, minimizes the patient's problem, and takes a negative stance toward the treatment program can seriously threaten a patient's chances for recovery. Parental alcohol or drug use will also have a significant impact on the adolescent's treatment. This underscores the importance of conducting a thorough clinical assessment of all immediate family members with regard to their drug/alcohol use, their attitudes toward the patient's problem, their attitudes toward the patient's treatment, and their overall level of psychosocial functioning. As discussed in Chapter 10, family members should be encouraged (or required) to participate in family groups that educate them about addictive disease, recovery, enabling, co-dependency, etc., that allow them to ventilate negative feelings such as anger, frustration, and guilt, and that provide advice, guidance, and support for dealing with the adolescent's behavior.

It is a mistake to assume that all adolescent cocaine addicts come from dysfunctional families and that the adolescent's cocaine use is merely a symptom of that dysfunction. Even when it is clear that there is family dysfunction and psychopathology that long predated the adolescent's drug use, it is best to address most of the parents' concerns in terms of their current reactions to the adolescent's problem rather than focusing on the underlying or historical cause. Otherwise, the guilt and defensiveness elicited in parents by provocative ventures into family etiology can make effective clinical management of the situation impossible. This does not mean, however, that parents should be absolved of the responsibility for dealing with the current crisis in their family and allowed to put the whole problem in the clinician's lap. They, too, must be willing to make significant changes in their attitude and behavior as an integral part of the overall treatment effort.

MISTRUST

Adolescents understandably regard the clinician as a parental authority figure and agent of their parents who will take sides against them. Mistrust, testing, and guardedness must be expected. The clinician's task is to convince the adolescent through consistent actions rather than words that he/she will be a supportive advocate and a nonjudgmental limit-setter without becoming an enabler. Complete confidentiality on all personal matters is promised, with the exception of any future drug use or other dangerously destructive behavior.

The challenge in treating adolescents is to simultaneously and delicately balance the needs to (1) establish a therapeutic alliance with the adolescent; (2) set appropriate limits and avoid being an enabler; (3) deal with the parents' desire to know the details of their adolescent's past and present drug use and their wish to have the problem "fixed" as quickly as possible; and (4) remain sensitive to any unacknowledged and/or unconscious jealousy and anger parents may have about the "private" communicative relationship developing between the therapist and their son or daughter. While there is no easy solution to this dilemma, it can be helpful to assign different therapists to the adolescent and to the family. This minimizes problems of split loyalty and breaches of confidentiality and gives both parties their own ally.

URINE TESTING

Taking supervised urine samples at least twice per week is a standard feature of the adolescent's treatment plan. If the patient misses a scheduled session and cannot come in the next day for a urine test, the parents should be asked to obtain a supervised urine sample at home in order to avoid gaps in the urine-testing schedule that could give the adolescent room for undetected drug use. When the program's urine-testing policy is explained at the beginning of treatment and incorporated into the signed treatment contract, few adolescents actually refuse to comply. Parents are often greatly relieved when their drug-abusing son/daughter is placed on urine surveillance because it frees them from the anxiety and uncertainty of not knowing for sure whether the adolescent is using drugs and of being constantly on guard for behavioral signs of drug use.

CHANGING FRIENDS

Since peer relationships are so central to the life of adolescents, it is unrealistic to expect that they will instantaneously give up their drugs and their friends upon entering a program. Adolescents should be cautioned about the dangers of spending time with drug-using friends, but should not be rigidly forbidden to have contact with them as a precondition of participating in the treatment program. It usually doesn't take long for adolescents to come to realize that being in contact with certain people makes it difficult, if not impossible, for them to stay drug free.

DEVELOPMENTAL ARREST

In general, the longer that adolescents have used cocaine or other drugs on a regular basis, the more severely their psychological growth and maturation have been arrested. It is difficult to complete the normal developmental tasks of adolescence while using drugs that alter brain chemistry and obliterate feelings. Adolescent drug abusers are often sorely lacking in their ability to recognize, label, and respond appropriately to feelings. Because they have existed in a chemically altered state during a critical period of maturational development, they often lack coping skills and have no stable sense of self. When they stop using drugs they lose the chemical buffer between themselves and reality. This can release a flood of unexpected and unfamiliar feelings for which the adolescent is ill-prepared. Moreover, the everyday experiences and interactions that used to be handled routinely under cocaine "anesthesia" now elicit strong feelings of hurt, disappointment, anger, frustration, boredom, nervousness, etc. Learning to anticipate and endure these feelings without using chemicals is essential to the adolescent's recovery.

Parents must be helped to accept that a drug-free adolescent is still an adolescent, subject to normal, albeit unpleasant, bouts of turmoil and conflict. Parents must not harbor unrealistic expectations that all of the adolescent's problems will vanish when the drug use stops. Teenagers are known to be moody, rebellious, unpredictable, secretive, sarcastic, and resistant to external control. Parents must also be helped to understand that their newly abstinent adolescent still needs limits, as well as a degree of freedom and independence and an opportunity to regain trust through consistent and responsible behavior.

GROUP THERAPY

Nearly all adolescent cocaine addicts should be treated in groups with other recovering adolescents. Group therapy is effective and appealing to teenage substance abusers because:

(1) peer relationships are so central to their lives;
(2) they will easily accept peer advice and identify with peer experiences;
(3) the group addresses both drug-use issues and their common age-related concerns;

(4) adolescents usually feel more protected and trusting when treated
with other adolescents rather than alone or with their families;

(5) groups provide an alternative socialization experience where adolescents can receive realistic feedback and have honest, nonexploit-
ive relationships with peers;

(6) newly abstinent adolescents need peer support to counteract the
boredom and loneliness they experience after giving up drugs;

(7) they need a buffer against the social ostracism and rejection from
friends who are contemptuous of their attempts to be drug free.

Group treatment may be contraindicated for those teens with serious coexisting psychiatric illnesses, who may not be able to cope with groups where
there is a high level of confrontation and peer pressure.

DRUGS AND DRIVING

A sense of invulnerability and immortality is typical of adolescents and
especially characteristic of substance-abusing teens who somehow choose to
believe that the dangers associated with certain types of behavior will never
affect them. Driving while intoxicated is a perfectly terrifying example.
Parents and adolescents alike must be educated about the special dangers
associated with the "roller coaster" effect of combining drugs, such as cocaine and alcohol, with opposite effects on brain function. The adolescent
who attempts to drive after ingesting this combination of a powerful stimulant and a powerful depressant may be fully alert one minute and stuporous
the next. In light of the life-threatening consequences of this behavior, the
clinician must be firm in advising parents to make the adolescent's driving
privileges contingent upon producing drug-free urines and passing breatha-
lyzer tests, without exception. A period of at least 30 days of initial abstinence is advised before considering restoration of the adolescent's driving
privileges.

SEXUAL ISSUES

Cocaine use may be intimately connected to sexual behavior and/or the
sexual problems of those adolescents who have become dependent on the
drug. Those who have had sex only while high on cocaine or other drugs
experience intense anxiety about their ability to handle sexual feelings without drugs. Teenagers who have been promiscuous on cocaine, especially
females, often need help with feelings of guilt, shame, and a diminished
sense of self-worth. Similarly, those who have engaged in homosexual acts
while under the influence of cocaine, despite being otherwise heterosexual,
may be terrified of being discovered and plagued with anxiety about their
sexual identity. Adolescent cocaine users, like adult users, may have engaged

in one or more types of sexually compulsive behaviors while intoxicated such as voyeurism, exhibitionism, multiple sexual encounters with unknown partners, excessive masturbation, and cross-dressing.

All of these issues make clear the importance of fully assessing the adolescent's sexual behavior and level of functioning before, during, and after involvement with cocaine. Because the topic of sexuality can be difficult to broach with adolescents, and especially so when the patient and therapist are of opposite sex, it is usually preferable for adolescents to be treated by same-sex therapists whenever possible. It is also advisable for adolescents to participate in a same-sex therapy group, as a supplement to their usual coed group, where they can more comfortably discuss sensitive topics and have an opportunity to benefit from more intensive contact with same-sex role models among peers and leaders in the group.

MEDICATION

None of the experimental pharmacologic treatments currently being tested in adult cocaine addicts has been tested for safety or effectiveness in adolescent cocaine addicts. Moreover, considering the unimpressive and inconsistent findings in adults thus far, routine administration of medication is entirely unjustified. However, no patient (adolescent or adult) who suffers from a serious psychiatric disorder should be deprived of potentially lifesaving nonaddictive psychotropic medication (such as antidepressants and antipsychotics) when such pharmacotherapy is medically indicated and appropriate.

WOMEN

There is no convincing evidence that the reasons why people use cocaine or the strategies for successfully treating those who become addicted differ greatly depending on gender. However, women's drug histories and drug-related problems are somewhat different from men's. Most of these differences stem from the traditionally different ways that they have been socialized and acculturated. But the "gender gap" has been closing in recent years as women have sought career opportunities and gained other rights and privileges similar to those of men. Along the way they have unavoidably acquired additional sources of stress as well, a factor that may be contributing to the increasing rates of substance abuse among today's women.

Treatment Considerations

The treatment strategies discussed in previous chapters are generally applicable to both women and men. For all cocaine addicts, both male and female, treatment must focus on abstinence, recovery, and relapse prevention. Psychological issues, some of which are inevitably gender-related, can and should be addressed in the course of treatment, but only after stable abstinence has been achieved. Some of the special considerations that commonly emerge in the treatment of female cocaine addicts are outlined below.

MALE SUPPLY SOURCES

Women cocaine addicts often receive "free" drugs from male companions, including spouses, lovers, friends, co-workers, and casual acquaintances. Sometimes women exchange sexual "favors" for cocaine, although during active addiction this type of bartering for drugs may not be consciously planned or conceived of as such. At the beginning of treatment, giving up cocaine may mean giving up all forms of contact with certain men. Some women must be helped to separate either temporarily or permanently from a spouse, live-in boyfriend, or habitual sexual partner who continues to use drugs. Even in cases where the relationship is obviously and seriously destructive, women may be so resistant to leaving that only an interim separation can be made to alleviate a crisis at the outset of treatment. Staying with a close drug-free friend or relative for a few days can lend some perspective on the relationship and make it easier for the woman surrounded by her mate's drug use to stop using cocaine. Peer support from other recovering women in the program, especially those who have been through similar experiences, can enhance a new patient's ability to cope with this problem.

CO-DEPENDENCY ISSUES

In a very real sense, most if not all women in our society are taught and encouraged to be co-dependents, i.e., to be nonassertive and nonaggressive, to put the needs of others before their own, to attend to and solve the problems of others instead of their own, to never say or do anything that would offend or inconvenience others, to make sacrifices for others above and beyond the call of duty, and to never get angry, resentful, or upset about any of this. Sometimes this co-dependency takes the form of trying to save an addict, sometimes it takes the form of becoming a cocaine addict in an effort to preserve relationships at all costs, even at the expense of self-care.

Many women of the 1980s find themselves trapped in an impossible bind, the "superwoman syndrome," trying to satisfy the often excessive and conflicting role demands of being a good mate, sex partner, professional, mother, daughter, sister, etc., all at the same time. Women who find it impossible to perfectly satisfy all of these role demands often fault themselves rather than the no-win situation produced by the unrealistic expectations placed upon them by others and by themselves. This can lead to a sense of inadequacy, to diminished competence, and ultimately to depression and despair.

Cocaine can temporarily supply the overworked and overstressed woman who is "running on empty" with energy, sexuality, elevated moods, and an illusion that everything is going just fine. Cocaine can obliterate problems from consciousness and supplant negative self-messages with positive ones. Paradoxically, women who strive for independence and self-confidence, feelings they derive artificially from cocaine, become intensely dependent on both the drug and the men who supply it to them in the process.

Obviously, learning to recognize and cope with these problems without using cocaine must be part of early treatment efforts with patients who are suffering with co-dependent "superwoman" issues. It is essential to reframe the patient's habitual need to satisfy others as admirable, but futile and self-destructive in its extreme. Sometimes it can be very difficult to get cocaine-addicted women to acknowledge needs and problems of their own, let alone give themselves sufficient priority, especially if their mates are also addicts. Women addicts are usually more concerned with their mate's recovery and making sure that he gets what he needs than they are with getting what they need for themselves. A women's co-dependency group (led by female therapists and counselors) that supplements participation in a primary coed recovery group is an excellent forum in which to address and overcome these problems.

EATING DISORDERS

Cocaine's appetite-suppressing effect has special appeal for women who want to lose weight. Women who are obsessed with their body image and prone to gross distortions about it, the hallmarks of eating disorders such as bulimia and anorexia, are often malignantly attracted to cocaine. The addictive thinking and behavior associated with binge eating can closely mimic that of a cocaine binge. The sense of competence and control derived from obsessively controlling one's food and caloric intake is remarkably parallel to that derived from using cocaine. Similarly, binge eating is used as a way to avoid rather than address emotional stresses and problems.

Cocaine-addicted women who have a history of eating disorders prior to and/or in combination with cocaine use can be expected to show an exacerbation or return of eating problems during abstinence from cocaine. It is essential that the eating problem not be ignored in favor of dealing with the cocaine problem exclusively. Abstinence from cocaine is the first priority, but the patient's eating disorder must be carefully monitored and specific treatment should be rendered expeditiously, including hospitalization if needed. Many patients with a history of serious eating disorders have received prior treatment for this problem and are in a state of partial recovery from it when they enter treatment for cocaine addiction. When possible, special groups for dually addicted women are strongly advised. Comprehensive diagnosis and treatment for eating disorders is important and should be provided by clinicians with special expertise in this area.

DEPRESSION

Depressive disorders are more common among women than men. Since initial cocaine use alleviates depression and chronic use creates or exacerbates it, women may be both especially susceptible to cocaine addiction and especially prone to developing severe depressions as a result of compulsive cocaine use. The importance of conducting an accurate psychiatric assessment of female patients that is uncomplicated by concurrent or recent drug use cannot be overemphasized here. After several weeks of cocaine abstinence, women who continue to show clear-cut depressive symptomatology may be candidates for a trial on antidepressants. As always, patients who receive such medications should be informed that the medication is for treatment of their depressive disorder, not their cocaine addiction, lest they develop false and potentially self-defeating hopes that the medication will permanently eliminate their desire for drugs.

COUPLES ISSUES

Women who enter treatment for cocaine addiction are almost always in the throes of serious relationship problems with a spouse or mate who may or may not be an addict himself. The problems are often due to a combination of drug-induced problems and other interpersonal conflicts that either existed before the drug use or emerge shortly after the drug use stops. Frequently, when the woman stops using cocaine the dynamics of the relationship change significantly. In cases of a "cocaine romance," an alliance that revolves almost entirely around cocaine, stopping the drug use may make it very clear to one or both parties that there is really no real relationship left to continue. On the other hand, in cases where a meaningful bond does exist between mates, there is a variety of common problems that arise which, if left unattended to, lead to increased discord and stress that inevitably exacerbate a newly abstinent woman's relapse potential.

Couples therapy conducted either in groups or with a single pair where one or both partners are drug addicts addresses a myriad of problems, including:

(1) dysfunctional interaction patterns;
(2) communication problems;
(3) role conflicts;
(4) sexual problems;

(5) parenting problems;
(6) money problems;
(7) anger and mistrust;
(8) power, control, and personal boundary issues;
(9) difficulties in expressing feelings of closeness and intimacy.

Couples groups can be extremely effective for many of the same reasons that groups are useful in other contexts: They provide role models, social support, and learning opportunities, and strengthen the identity and commitment of the couple as an adult pair seeking greater stability in their relationship. Couples groups should be limited to no more than three or four pairs and are best led by male-female co-therapy teams. This arrangement gives group members an opportunity to identify with a same-sex leader and to simultaneously benefit from observing the interaction between the opposite-sex leaders, who serve as a model "couple" communicating effectively with one another and conveying mutual respect.

HEALTH-CARE PROFESSIONALS

Serious drug abuse among the ranks of health-care professionals is certainly not a new phenomenon, but cocaine has probably infiltrated this subgroup to a much greater extent than any other illegal drug, with the possible exception of marijuana. Since drug abuse is an occupational hazard among physicians, nurses, pharmacists, dentists and other professionals who have enhanced access to drugs, it is a cause for serious public and professional concern.

There is continuing disagreement about the true incidence of drug addiction among medical and mental health professionals and whether the risks of becoming addicted are any higher for this subgroup than for the population at large. In addition to some of the more obvious contributors to this addiction risk, including the stressful and demanding nature of a professional career where one is responsible for the health and well-being of others coupled with easy access to a wide variety of psychoactive prescription drugs, the health-care professions are currently replete with individuals who fit the rather typical demographic profile of a large segment of the adult cocaine-using population. This profile includes people who are between the ages of 25 and 45, employed, middle-class, reasonably well-educated, and success-oriented, who earn good incomes, have a history of using marijuana or other drugs at least occasionally as teenagers or young adults, and have a history of reasonably stable functioning with no serious psychiatric illness or previous addiction to other drugs.

Thus, the increased incidence of drug abuse among health-care professionals may be due primarily to the same sociocultural trends that have made drug abuse a problem throughout the American workplace: namely, that the "baby boomers" have grown up and taken their drug-receptive attitudes and drug-oriented lifestyles into the workplace, including the health-care professions. Whether health-care professionals are seemingly at greater risk as an artifact of demographics or because of certain psychological factors common to people who enter this type of work, the treatment of cocaine-addicted health-care professionals poses a number of special problems.

Treatment Considerations

CONFIDENTIALITY VS. CONSUMER PROTECTION

One of the major dilemmas for clinicians treating addicted health-care professionals involves balancing the patient's needs for confidentiality with consumers' need for protection from the potentially harmful or even life-threatening behavior of an impaired practitioner. Many cocaine-addicted health-care professionals avoid seeking treatment in the first place because of fears about possible career repercussions if the problem is exposed. Thus, threatening to immediately report the patient to professional licensing/misconduct boards at the very outset of treatment is of little value and distinctly antithetical to the all-important initial goal of establishing a therapeutic alliance with the patient. Yet the clinician must carefully guard against becoming an enabler of the patient's continued cocaine use.

One way to solve this dilemma is to formulate a treatment contract with the patient that stipulates the following requirements, in addition to the usual ones:

(1) The patient will voluntarily discontinue all professional activities until at least one week of total abstinence from cocaine and all other mood-altering chemicals is achieved, verified by urine testing.
(2) The patient will voluntarily discontinue all professional activities during any subsequent periods of relapse.
(3) The patient will voluntarily enter a residential program at such time that the clinician deems this action to be necessary.
(4) The patient gives the clinician written authorization to report his/her cocaine problem to the appropriate professional organizations and/or regulatory agencies if the patient drops out of treatment prematurely, against the clinician's advice, or fails to comply with any other stipulation of the contract.

This arrangement sets appropriate limits on dangerous behavior which could result from any further use of cocaine.

Some health-care professionals come to treatment having already been reported to the authorities by an employer, family member, or colleague. In these cases, patients are usually required by law to complete a treatment program in order to maintain their professional license or to have it reinstated. Their activities are usually monitored by an impaired professionals committee which stipulates certain minimum requirements concerning length and type of treatment, frequency of supervised urine screens, attendance at self-help meetings, etc., that must be met to avoid further consequences to their licensure status. Since most health-care professionals highly value their careers and have a history of being able to function well before cocaine addiction, their prognosis in treatment is usually very good.

ASSUMING THE PATIENT ROLE

Many addicted professionals have difficulty with the unavoidable role reversal they must face upon entering treatment. They are accustomed to being the doctor, not the patient. Their difficulty accepting the patient role may manifest itself in at least several ways. They may talk about themselves in a very intellectualized clinical manner, offering professional opinions and diagnoses about their own behavior and the behavior of others. They may be overly critical of the therapist's clinical judgment and technique, demanding explanations and rationales for his/her every move. They may attempt to "pull rank" on the therapist in an area where they have special knowledge. They may relate to the therapist in an overly informal, friendly manner so as to negate the professional aspects of the relationship. They may demand special favors not granted to other patients, such as telephone privileges, special appointment times, and a place to wait other than the waiting room.

These difficulties must be handled in a thoughtful, respectful, face-saving manner that eases the addicted professional into accepting the unfamiliar role of being the recipient rather than the provider of professional treatment services. An initial period of intensive individual counseling may be needed to help those practitioners who are especially frightened and anxious work through their reluctance to accept the patient role. Where possible, addicted health-care professionals should be placed in recovery groups that contain others with whom they can identify. Yet, creating homogeneous groups of recovering physicians or other health-care professionals may not be the best arrangement, for the same reason that restricting groups exclusively to cocaine addicts is not optimal: It perpetuates a sense of elitism, uniqueness, and exemption that can be a major obstacle to recovery. Professionals' concerns about jeopardizing their anonymity in mixed groups generally subside once they reach the point of accepting that they are addicted, that their problem is really no different from that of other addicts, and that these others also have much to lose by public exposure.

PROFESSIONAL ATHLETES

The use of cocaine by professional athletes has generated increasing attention and public concern in recent years. Public outrage about drug use in professional sports rises out of a collective sense that athletes who use illegal drugs are betraying the public's confidence and trust. There is an unspoken contract that these extraordinarily high-paid performers should maintain themselves in the best possible physical condition and be good role models for the millions of youngsters who idolize them.

The percentage of athletes in professional sports who use cocaine may be no greater than among the population at large, but when an athlete's drug use is exposed the revelation becomes a highly publicized media event. It is often assumed that athletes use cocaine to improve their athletic performance, but in fact this is rarely the case. When athletes use cocaine, they almost always do so during their time off—after or between games, not before or during them. Their initial introduction to cocaine is likely to occur in a social situation—a party or other social gathering. They use the drug primarily for its euphorigenic mood-altering effects, and perhaps only incidentally for its short-lived energizing properties. To use cocaine during a game for its performance-enhancing effects, an athlete would have to retire to the locker room every half-hour or so to snort a few lines, otherwise he would not be able to maintain the high and postpone the crash. Those who smoke freebase or crack would not be inclined even to think about performing athletically while high on the drug, let alone actually attempt to do so.

Certain characteristics of professional athletes and the position they occupy in our society probably put them at increased risk for cocaine addiction and also make them more difficult to treat. In many ways, professional athletes can become victims of their own success. Most have lived very sheltered lives. Achieving prominence when young and often psychologically immature, they may become tragically suspended in a state of perpetual adolescence fostered by an entourage of people who enable them. They are purposefully shielded from the normal intrusions of the real world so as to not distract them from the task of maintaining superlative athletic performance. This artificial reality sometimes deprives them of acquiring even the most basic life-management skills, such as paying household bills or parking tickets and balancing a checkbook.

Quite naturally, these athletes become accustomed to special treatment and develop a sense of entitlement and invulnerability. They become extraordinarily image conscious. Celebrity, wealth, and adulation can be intoxicating. It is not difficult to become enamored with life in the fast lane. Cocaine fits right in with all of this, seems like a perfect drug, and is offered without their even asking. When a star player is using cocaine, the coach and other team personnel may know it but hesitate to challenge or confront him. Their concerns for the player are sometimes overriden by fears about negative publicity and losing games if a key player is suspended or goes into a treatment program because of cocaine use.

Treatment Considerations

Few cocaine-addicted athletes seek treatment voluntarily. Their motivation to enter a program comes almost entirely out of the desire to avoid loss of career and income. When professional athletes are finally brought to treatment, their insistence on special concessions and exemptions from the program rules can pose immediate difficulties. They may insist on maintaining their celebrity status by relating to other patients as their fans rather than their peers. This posture is reinforced when the athlete's fellow patients ask for autographs or complimentary tickets to games and keep the focus of their interaction on sports rather than recovery.

Probably the most serious obstacle to successful treatment is the athlete's schedule, which can make continuity between sessions virtually impossible. During the playing season athletes are almost always involved in playing or preparing for a game at home or on the road. The cooperation of the patient's coach is essential in making sure that appropriate priority is given to attending therapy sessions and self-help meetings, whenever possible.

Guidelines for the clinician treating professional athletes include the following:

(1) The athlete's contact with counselors and self-help meetings in different cities must be arranged and coordinated.
(2) When face-to-face counseling sessions are impossible, telephone sessions with the primary therapist should be conducted on a regular basis and supervised urine samples should be taken from the athlete by team personnel at least twice every week.
(3) The athlete's coach should be involved in the treatment similar to that for family members, wherever possible. The coach should be educated about addiction, recovery, treatment, and co-dependency. Many coaches exhibit serious co-dependency problems, including destructive enabling of the cocaine-addicted athlete, which is fueled by the financial pressures on them to win games at all cost.

(4) The athlete's atypical life circumstances should be taken into account, but special concessions that undermine his treatment and reinforce his sense of entitlement should be categorically avoided.

(5) With assistance from the coach, the athlete should designate a fellow team member (someone who does not use drugs) to be available for support and encouragement, especially at night or during other unstructured times when not working. This person must be made fully aware of the patient's problem and, if possible, meet with the therapist for basic guidance and orientation about how to be most helpful.

(6) Other patients in the program should be asked to treat the athlete and all other patients, regardless of social status, as recovering peers rather than stars and be told why this is so important. Behavior that is observed to be inconsistent with this request should be discouraged.

Final Comment

THE MAJOR THRUST of this book has been to describe techniques for treating cocaine addiction successfully. An effort has been made to present practical suggestions and specific guidelines, wherever possible, in order to maximize the usefulness of this material to front-line clinicians, program administrators, family members of cocaine addicts, and to cocaine addicts themselves, all of whom are likely to benefit (either personally or professionally) from a more detailed knowledge of the treatment process.

The treatment of cocaine addiction is one of the most critical issues in the chemical dependency treatment field today. Hopefully, the information, ideas, and suggestions presented in this book not only expand current knowledge about treatment, but also point the way to promising new developments in the future.

Appendices

Cocaine Assessment Profile (CAP)

I. *COCAINE USE*

1. How long ago did you first try cocaine? _____
2. How did you use it the first time?
   _____ snort _____ freebase _____ i.v.
3. How long did you use cocaine on an "occasional" basis before your use became regular and intensified? _____
4. Have you ever freebased? _____ Yes _____ No
5. Have you ever injected cocaine? _____ Yes _____ No
6. Currently, what is your usual method of use?
   _____ snort _____ freebase _____ i.v.
7. On average, how many grams of cocaine do you use per week?
   _____ grams
8. How much money do you spend on cocaine per week? $_____ per week
9. On average, how many days per week do you use cocaine? _____ days
10. Do you tend to go on "binges"? _____ Yes _____ No
    If yes, how long does the binge usually last? _____ days
    How many grams do you use during a typical binge? _____ grams

11. In what types of situations do you usually use cocaine? (Check all that apply).

    _____ alone   _____ at home
    _____ with friends   _____ at parties
    _____ with spouse/mate   _____ at work
    _____ with other sexual partner

12. During what portion of the day do you usually use cocaine? (Check all that apply).

    _____ morning   _____ afternoon   _____ evening   _____ late night

13. Since you first started using cocaine on a regular basis, what is the longest time you've been able to stop completely? _____

14. Check below any *physical* problems caused by your cocaine use:

    _____ Low energy   _____ Hepatitis
    _____ Sleep problems   _____ Other infections
    _____ Hands tremble   _____ Heart "flutters"
    _____ Runny nose   _____ Nausea
    _____ Nasal sores, bleeding   _____ Chills
    _____ Sinus congestion   _____ Seizures with loss of consciousness
    _____ Headaches   _____ Excessive weight loss
    _____ Cough, sore throat   _____ Other (describe) _____
    _____ Chest congestion   _____
    _____ Black phlegm

15. Check below any negative effects of cocaine on your *mood or mental state*:

    _____ Irritable   _____ Paranoia
    _____ Short-tempered   _____ Anxiety/nervousness
    _____ Depression   _____ Panic attacks
    _____ Memory problems   _____ Suicidal impulses
    _____ Loss of sex drive   _____ Violent impulses
    _____ Other (please describe) _____
    _____

16. Check any negative effects of cocaine on your *relationships* with other people:

    _____ Caused arguments with spouse/mate
    _____ Spouse/mate has threatened to leave
    _____ Caused relationship to break up
    _____ Became socially isolated and withdrawn
    _____ Harmed sexual relationship
    _____ Harmed ability to talk openly and honestly with others

17. Check any negative effects of cocaine use on your *work or studies*:

_____ Come late to work/school   _____ Spend too much time on breaks
_____ Miss days of work/shcool   _____ Harmed relationship with boss
_____ Reduced productivity at   _____ Got fired from a job
     work/school
_____ Other (please describe) _____

_____

18. Check any negative effects of cocaine use on your *financial situation*:

_____ Used up all money in bank   _____ Unable to keep up with bills
_____ Gotten in debt   _____ No extra money
_____ Other (please describe) _____

_____

19. Check any legal consequences of your cocaine use:
_____ Arrested for possession or sale of cocaine
_____ Arrested for other crime(s) related to cocaine sale/use

20. Has your cocaine use caused you to:

_____ Have a car accident   _____ Physically hurt someone
_____ Have a physical fight   _____ Attempt suicide
     with someone   _____ Deal drugs
_____ Have an unwanted sexual   _____ Steal from work, family
     encounter   or friends

II. OTHER DRUG USE

1. Have you *ever* used any of the following substances?

Marijuana	_____ Yes	_____ No
Amphetamines	_____ Yes	_____ No
LSD or other psychedelics	_____ Yes	_____ No
Valium or other tranquilizers	_____ Yes	_____ No
Barbiturates	_____ Yes	_____ No
Quaaludes	_____ Yes	_____ No
Heroin	_____ Yes	_____ No
Other opiates	_____ Yes	_____ No
Alcohol	_____ Yes	_____ No
Cigarettes/nicotine	_____ Yes	_____ No

2. Check below any substances you are currently using (within past 30 days) and indicate how much and how often you use each one:

	How much	*How often*
_Marijuana		
_Amphetamines		
_LSD/other psychedelics		

	How much	*How often*
__Tranquilizers (Valium, etc.)	_____	_____
__Sleeping pills (barbiturates)	_____	_____
__Quaaludes	_____	_____
__Heroin	_____	_____
__Other opiates	_____	_____
__Alcohol	_____	_____
__Cigarettes/nicotine	_____	_____

3. Do you currently feel dependent on any of these substances?
   _____ Yes _____ No.   If yes, please explain: _____

4. Have you ever had a problem with any of these substances in the past? _____ Yes _____ No. If yes, please describe: _____

5. Have you ever used any of these substances on a regular basis for one month or longer? _____ Yes _____ No. If yes, please describe _____

6. Are you currently taking any prescription medication? _____ Yes _____ No   If yes, please describe and give physician's name and reason for use: _____

III. *TREATMENT FOR DRUG OR ALCOHOL ABUSE*

1. Have you ever been in treatment for drug or alcohol abuse?
   _____ Yes _____ No   If yes, please describe below:

	Name of program	
Dates of treatment:	hospital, doctor:	Type of treatment:

2. Have you ever attended AA, NA, CA or other self-help group meetings? _____ Yes _____ No.   If yes, please give dates of attendance:

Cocaine Addiction Severity Test (CAST)

Please answer yes or no to each question below. Do not leave any questions unanswered.

	YES	NO
1. Do you have trouble turning down cocaine when it is offered to you?	___	___
2. Do you tend to use up whatever supplies of cocaine you have on hand even though you try to save some for another time?	___	___
3. Have you been trying to stop using cocaine but find that somehow you always go back to it?	___	___
4. Do you go on cocaine binges for 24 hours or longer?	___	___
5. Do you need to be high on cocaine in order to have a good time?	___	___
6. Are you afraid that you will be bored or unhappy without cocaine?	___	___
7. Are you afraid that you will be less able to function without cocaine?	___	___
8. Does the sight, thought or mention of cocaine trigger urges and cravings for the drug?	___	___

	YES	NO
9. Are you sometimes preoccupied with thoughts about cocaine?	—	—
10. Do you sometimes feel an irresistable compulsion to use cocaine?	—	—
11. Do you feel psychologically addicted to cocaine?	—	—
12. Do you feel guilty and ashamed of using cocaine and like yourself less for doing it?	—	—
13. Have you been spending less time with "straight" people since you've been using more cocaine?	—	—
14. Are you frightened by the strength of your cocaine habit?	—	—
15. Do you tend to spend time with certain people or go to certain places because you know that cocaine will be available?	—	—
16. Do you use cocaine at work?	—	—
17. Do people tell you that your behavior or personality has changed even though they might not know it's due to drugs?	—	—
18. Has cocaine led you to abuse alcohol or other drugs?	—	—
19. Do you ever drive a car while high on cocaine, alcohol, or other drugs?	—	—
20. Have you ever neglected any significant responsibilities at home or at work due to cocaine use?	—	—
21. Have your values and priorities been distorted by cocaine use?	—	—
22. Do you deal cocaine in order to support your own use?	—	—
23. Would you be using even more cocaine if you had more money to spend on it or otherwise had greater access to the drug?	—	—
24. Do you hide your cocaine use from straight friends or family because you're afraid of their reactions?	—	—
25. Have you become less interested in health-promoting activities (e.g. exercise, sports, diet, etc.) due to cocaine use?	—	—
26. Have you become less involved in your job or career due to cocaine use?	—	—
27. Do you find yourself lying and making excuses because of cocaine use?	—	—

	YES	NO
28. Do you tend to deny and downplay the severity of your cocaine problem?	—	—
29. Have you been unable to stop using cocaine even though you know that it is having negative effects on your life?	—	—
30. Has cocaine use jeopardized your job or career?	—	—
31. Do you worry whether you are capable of living a normal and satisfying life without cocaine?	—	—
32. Are you having financial problems due to cocaine use?	—	—
33. Are you having problems with your spouse or mate due to cocaine use?	—	—
34. Has cocaine use had negative effects on your physical health?	—	—
35. Is cocaine having a negative effect on your mood or mental state?	—	—
36. Has your sexual functioning been disrupted by cocaine use?	—	—
37. Have you become less sociable due to cocaine use?	—	—
38. Have you missed days of work due to cocaine use?	—	—
Total	—	—

APPENDIX C

Sexual Compulsions Questionnaire

1. Does your drug use at times lead to sexual fantasies or behavior?
   Yes _____ No _____
2. What percentage of the time would you say your drug use is combined with sexual fantasies or behavior? _____

   _____

3. Do you find that any of the following behaviors are part of your drug experience? (Please check those that apply)

   _____ Excessive masturbation
   _____ Excessive intercourse
   _____ Porno movies
   _____ Peep shows
   _____ Exhibitionism
   _____ Voyeurism
   _____ Sado masochistic sex
   _____ Cross dressing
   _____ Frequenting prostitutes
   _____ Obsessive sexual thoughts and fantasies

4. Are any of the above a problem for you?
   Yes _____ No _____
   Please explain _____

   _____

5. Were any of the above a problem prior to your drug use?
Yes _____ No _____
6. If you answered yes to question 5 has the problem become worse since you began using drugs? Yes _____ No _____
Please explain _____
_____

7. Is it common for you to be involved in several intimate relationships at one time? Yes _____ No _____
8. Are you currently or have you ever been preoccupied with thoughts of a person to the point that it interferes with your daily activities?
Yes _____ No _____
Please explain _____
_____
_____

The South Oaks Gambling Screen

1. Please indicate which of the following types of gambling you have done in your lifetime. For each type, mark one answer: "not at all," "less than once a week," or "once a week or more."

	Not at all	Less than once a week	Once a week or more	
a.	___	___	___	played cards for money
b.	___	___	___	bet on horses, dogs, or other animals (in off-track betting, at the track, or with a bookie)
c.	___	___	___	bet on sports (parlay cards, with a bookie, or at jai alai)
d.	___	___	___	played dice games (including craps, over and under, or other dice games) for money
e.	___	___	___	went to casino (legal or otherwise)
f.	___	___	___	played the numbers or bet on lotteries
g.	___	___	___	played bingo
h.	___	___	___	played the stock and/or commodities market
i.	___	___	___	played slot machines, poker machines, or other gambling machines

j. ___ ___ ___ bowled, shot pool, played golf, or played some other game of skill for money

2. What is the largest amount of money you have ever gambled with on any one day?
   ___ never have gambled
   ___ $1 or less
   ___ more than $1 up to $10
   ___ more than $10 up to $100
   ___ more than $100 up to $1,000
   ___ more than $1,000 up to $10,000
   ___ more than $10,000

3. Do (did) your parents have a gambling problem?
   ___ both my father and mother gamble (or gambled) too much
   ___ my father gambles (or gambled) too much
   ___ my mother gambles (or gambled) too much
   ___ neither one gambles (or gambled) too much

4. When you gamble, how often do you go back another day to win back money you lost?
   ___ never
   ___ some of the time (less than half the time) I lost
   ___ most of the time I lost
   ___ every time I lost

5. Have you ever claimed to be winning money gambling but weren't really? In fact, you lost?
   ___ never (or never gamble)
   ___ yes, less than half the time I lost
   ___ yes, most of the time

6. Do you feel you have ever had a problem with gambling?
   ___ no
   ___ yes, in the past, but not now
   ___ yes

7. Did you ever gamble more than you intended to? ☐ Yes ☐ No

8. Have people criticized your gambling? ☐ Yes ☐ No

9. Have you ever felt guilty about the way you gamble or what happens when you gamble? ☐ Yes ☐ No

10. Have you ever felt like you would like to stop gambling but didn't think you could? ☐ Yes ☐ No

11. Have you ever hidden betting slips, lottery tickets, gambling money, or other signs of gambling from your spouse, children, or other important people in your life? ☐ Yes ☐ No

12. Have you ever argued with people you live with over how you handle money? ☐ Yes ☐ No

13. (If you answered yes to question 12): Have money arguments ever centered on your gambling? ☐ Yes ☐ No

14. Have you ever borrowed from someone and not
    paid them back as a result of your gambling?   ☐ Yes   ☐ No
15. Have you ever lost time from work (or school)
    due to gambling?   ☐ Yes   ☐ No
16. If you borrowed money to gamble or to pay gambling debts, who or
    where did you borrow from? (check "yes" or "no" for each)
    a. from household money   ☐ Yes   ☐ No
    b. from your spouse   ☐ Yes   ☐ No
    c. from other relatives or in-laws   ☐ Yes   ☐ No
    d. from banks, loan companies, or credit unions   ☐ Yes   ☐ No
    e. from credit cards   ☐ Yes   ☐ No
    f. from loan sharks (Shylocks)   ☐ Yes   ☐ No
    g. you cashed in stocks, bonds, or other securities ☐ Yes   ☐ No
    h. you sold personal or family property   ☐ Yes   ☐ No
    i. you borrowed on your checking account
       (passed bad checks)   ☐ Yes   ☐ No
    j. you have (had) a credit line with a bookie   ☐ Yes   ☐ No
    k. you have (had) a credit line with a casino   ☐ Yes   ☐ No

Scores are determined by adding up the number of questions that show an
"at risk" response; one point for each.

Questions 1, 2, and 3 are not counted.   Question 12 not counted
_____ Question 4: most of the time I   _____ Question 13: yes
        lost, or every time I lost   _____ Question 14: yes
_____ Question 5: yes, less than half the   _____ Question 15: yes
        time I lost, or yes, most of the   _____ Question 16a: yes
        time   _____ Question 16b: yes
_____ Question 6: yes, in the past, but   _____ Question 16c: yes
        not now, or yes   _____ Question 16d: yes
_____ Question 7: yes   _____ Question 16e: yes
_____ Question 8: yes   _____ Question 16f: yes
_____ Question 9: yes   _____ Question 16g: yes
_____ Question 10: yes   _____ Question 16h: yes
_____ Question 11: yes   _____ Question 16i: yes
                                               Questions 16j and 16k not
                                               counted

Total = _____ (20 questions are counted)

Note: A score of 5 or more indicates probable pathological gambling.
      A score of 1-4 indicates the presence of some gambling-related problems.
This questionnaire was developed by Henry R. Lesieur and Sheila B. Blume (Lesieur and Blume,
1987). Courtesy of South Oaks Foundation.

Gambling Questionnaire

Please answer each question yes or no.

	YES	NO
1. Do you lose time from work due to gambling?	___	___
2. Is gambling making your home life unhappy?	___	___
3. Is gambling affecting your reputation?	___	___
4. Have you ever felt remorse after gambling?	___	___
5. Do you ever gamble to get money to pay debts or to otherwise solve other financial difficulties?	___	___
6. Does gambling decrease your ambition or efficiency?	___	___
7. After losing, do you feel you must return as soon as possible and win back your losses?	___	___
8. After a win, do you have a strong urge to return and win more?	___	___
9. Do you often gamble until your last dollar is gone?	___	___
10. Do you ever borrow to finance your gambling?	___	___
11. Have you ever sold any real or personal property to finance gambling?	___	___

	YES	NO
12. Are you reluctant to use "gambling money" for normal expenditures?	——	——
13. Does gambling make you careless of the welfare of your family?	——	——
14. Do you ever gamble longer than you had planned?	——	——
15. Do you ever gamble to escape worry or trouble?	——	——
16. Have you ever committed, or considered committing, an illegal act to finance gambling?	——	——
17. Does gambling cause you to have difficulty sleeping?	——	——
18. Do arguments, disappointments or frustrations give you an urge to gamble?	——	——
19. Do you have an urge to celebrate any good fortune by gambling?	——	——
20. Have you ever considered self-destruction as a result of your gambling?	——	——
21. Do you believe that lack of more money is your problem?	——	——
22. Do you expect an instantaneous cure for your problem?	——	——
23. Can you conceive of life without gambling?	——	——
24. Do you see payment of all your outstanding debts as the solution to your problem?	——	——
25. Do you expect to be bored, depressed, irritable, or anxious when you stop gambling?	——	——
26. Do you drink or use drugs before, during or after you gamble?	——	——
27. Do you promise your spouse or mate to stop gambling?	——	——
28. Are you away from home or unavailable to the family for long periods of time when you gamble?	——	——
29. Do you promise faithfully that you will stop gambling and beg for another chance, yet continue to gamble?	——	——
30. Has your personality changed as a result of continued gambling?	——	——
31. Are you addicted to the "action" and stimulation in gambling?	——	——

Eating Disorders Questionnaire

1. Have you ever suspected or been told that you have an eating problem?
   _____ Yes _____ No
   If yes, _____ bulimia?
   _____ anorexia?
   _____ compulsive overeating?
2. Do you go on food binges where you eat several meals worth of calories in one sitting? _____ Yes _____ No
   A. If yes, how often does this happen?_____
   B. Do you ever force yourself to vomit after an eating binge or take laxatives or diuretics? _____ Yes _____ No
   If yes, please explain _____

   C. Do you feel anxious and depressed after an eating binge? _____ Yes _____ No
   D. Have you tried to stop bingeing on your own without success? _____ Yes _____ No
   E. Since you first started bingeing on food, what's the longest time you've been able to abstain from bingeing? _____

3. Are you obsessed with your body proportions to the point where it dictates too much of your mental life? _____ Yes _____ No

4. Do you fear being unable to stop eating voluntarily? ＿＿＿ Yes ＿＿＿ No

5. Do you try to lose weight by fasting or "crash" diets? ＿＿＿ Yes ＿＿＿ No
   If yes, how often? ＿＿＿＿＿＿＿＿＿＿＿＿＿＿＿＿＿＿＿＿＿＿＿＿＿＿

6. Would you label yourself a "compulsive eater," one who engages in episodes of uncontrolled eating? ＿＿＿ Yes ＿＿＿ No

7. Are you generally terrified of gaining weight? ＿＿＿ Yes ＿＿＿ No

8. Are you preoccuppied with the desire to be thinner? ＿＿＿ Yes ＿＿＿ No

9. Are you chronically dissatisfied with your body weight or shape? ＿＿＿ Yes ＿＿＿ No

10. Do you binge and/or starve yourself in response to stress? ＿＿＿ Yes ＿＿＿ No

11. Do other people seem worried about your eating patterns and say that you have a problem with food? ＿＿＿ Yes ＿＿＿ No
    If yes, please explain ＿＿＿＿＿＿＿＿＿＿＿＿＿＿＿＿＿＿＿＿
    ＿＿＿＿＿＿＿＿＿＿＿＿＿＿＿＿＿＿＿＿＿＿＿＿＿＿＿＿＿＿＿＿

12. Have your unusual eating patterns caused you any medical problems? ＿＿＿ Yes ＿＿＿ No If yes, please explain ＿＿＿＿＿＿＿＿
    ＿＿＿＿＿＿＿＿＿＿＿＿＿＿＿＿＿＿＿＿＿＿＿＿＿＿＿＿＿＿＿＿

13. In what ways is your life at work and/or at home disrupted by your eating problems? ＿＿＿＿＿＿＿＿＿＿＿＿＿＿＿＿＿＿＿

14. Have you ever received formal treatment for an eating problem? ＿＿＿ Yes ＿＿＿ No If yes, please give details ＿＿＿＿＿＿＿＿
    ＿＿＿＿＿＿＿＿＿＿＿＿＿＿＿＿＿＿＿＿＿＿＿＿＿＿＿＿＿＿＿＿

15. Have you ever attended a self-help group or weight-loss program? ＿＿＿ Yes ＿＿＿ No If yes, please give details ＿＿＿＿＿＿＿
    ＿＿＿＿＿＿＿＿＿＿＿＿＿＿＿＿＿＿＿＿＿＿＿＿＿＿＿＿＿＿＿＿
    ＿＿＿＿＿＿＿＿＿＿＿＿＿＿＿＿＿＿＿＿＿＿＿＿＿＿＿＿＿＿＿＿

16. Have you ever used cocaine, amphetamines, diet pills, or other drugs to control your appetite? ＿＿＿ Yes ＿＿＿ No If yes, please give details ＿＿＿＿＿＿＿＿＿＿＿＿＿＿＿＿＿＿＿＿＿＿＿＿
    ＿＿＿＿＿＿＿＿＿＿＿＿＿＿＿＿＿＿＿＿＿＿＿＿＿＿＿＿＿＿＿＿
    ＿＿＿＿＿＿＿＿＿＿＿＿＿＿＿＿＿＿＿＿＿＿＿＿＿＿＿＿＿＿＿＿

17. If you stop using cocaine, do you expect to have problems with eating? ＿＿＿ Yes ＿＿＿ No

APPENDIX G

Relapse Attitude Inventory

Answer each question as follows:
"P" past problem, but not now
"C" current problem
"N" never a problem

_____ 1. Are you angry that you can't return to "controlled" drug/alcohol use again?

_____ 2. Are you resisting the idea of not drinking, or smoking marijuana even "occasionally"?

_____ 3. Are you being superficially compliant with the program and paying "lip service" to the advice you are receiving?

_____ 4. Are you making promises and commitments about actions you don't follow through on?

_____ 5. Are you failing to sever ties with drug-using friends, lovers, and acquaintances?

_____ 6. Are you holding onto the phone numbers of your dealers because you think you might possibly want to contact them again in the future?

_____ 7. Are you holding onto the notion that your dealer is your "friend"?

_____ 8. Are you serving as a contact, resource, or middleman in drug buys for others?

_____ 9. Do you allow others to get high in your home?

_____ 10. Have you failed to discard all drug paraphernalia and drug supplies?

_____ 11. Are you harboring a secret "stash" in your home, car, safe deposit vault, friend's home, or other secret hiding place?

_____ 12. If you thoroughly cleaned your home or car, would you "accidently" come across a drug supply you happened to forget about?

_____ 13. Do you feel that being in a treatment program means you're a loser?

_____ 14. Do you feel like a helpless victim of your addiction problem?

_____ 15. Are you immersed in self-pity about your addiction and repeatedly asking yourself "why me"?

_____ 16. Are you looking to your therapist for the "answers" to your addiction problem?

_____ 17. Are you blindly doing what you are told and nothing more?

_____ 18. Are you letting others take responsibility for your recovery?

_____ 19. Are you mechanically following the advice of others so that if it doesn't work out, you can blame your failure on them?

_____ 20. Are you telling others what they want to hear, attempting to keep them off your back?

_____ 21. Do you promise yourself or others that you will never get high again?

_____ 22. Are you hoping that being in treatment will give you the strength to return to controlled drug use again?

_____ 23. Do you believe you can put yourself in "high risk" situations without being tempted to get high?

_____ 24. Do you downplay or ignore the risks of being in contact with people, places, and things associated with your prior drug use?

_____ 25. Do you think that while some addicts may need the "crutch" of AA, CA, or NA, you don't need to rely on others for help?

_____ 26. Do you believe that a drink or a joint won't impede your recovery in any way?

_____ 27. Do you consider yourself to be better, smarter, or more "together" than everyone else in your program?

_____ 28. Do you consider some of the program rules simply not applicable to your particular situation?

_____ 29. Are you secretly planning to drop out of the program prematurely, hoping to make it on your own thereafter?

_____ 30. Do you "unavoidably" miss meetings or sessions because of schedule conflicts that could really be removed with a more honest effort on your part?

_____ 31. Do you consider AA, CA, or NA meetings as undignified, low class, or for losers?

_____ 32. Do you consider yourself as being intelligent enough to beat the odds and avoid relapse without following advice or making significant lifestyle changes?

_____ 33. Do you superficially accept the advice of your therapist and peers, but later discount what they say and fail to follow through with their suggestions?

_____ 34. Are you hoping to find another program or therapist to make recovery easier for you?

_____ 35. Do you think of your therapist and peers as rigid, narrow-minded, or unable to understand your special needs?

_____ 36. Are you secretly contemptuous of your therapist or peers?

_____ 37. Are you being manipulative and deceitful in order to avoid responsibility for your actions or the lack of them?

_____ 38. Are you determined to have a "perfect" recovery?

_____ 39. Are you hoping that your determination and willpower to be abstinent will result in a successful recovery?

_____ 40. Do you set impossible standards and expectations for yourself and others?

_____ 41. Do you continue to "romanticize" and glorify previous drug experiences?

_____ 42. Do you argue about insignificant things and insist on being right most of the time?

_____ 43. Do you tend to magnify difficulties and consider every problem a disaster?

_____ 44. Do you have trouble admitting faults and weaknesses?

_____ 45. Do you tend to blame your problems on others, especially those closest to you?

_____ 46. Do you attempt to make others feel guilty and defensive when they try to hold you accountable for your behavior?

_____ 47. Do you believe that recovery is just a matter of staying away from drugs and alcohol?

_____ 48. Are you focusing on someone else's recovery more than your own?

_____ 49. Are you generally being negative, blaming, and chronically dissatisfied?

_____ 50. Are you angry and disappointed because now that you've stopped using drugs, life still isn't going "just fine"?

_____ 51. Are you angry that the victims of your addiction are not granting you instant trust and forgiveness?

_____ 52. Are you secretly intending to cut down the frequency of your drug use without stopping it completely?

_____ 53. Do you believe it impossible to have a satisfying social or sex life without drugs or alcohol?

_____ 54. Do you feel like your recovery is a lonely endurance test?

_____ 55. Are you allowing boredom, stress, or other hassles to accumulate so you can justify a return to drugs as inevitable or as a well-deserved "treat" or "relief"?

_____ 56. Are you engaging in other addictive behaviors (compulsive gambling, eating, sexuality), but not mentioning these problems to your therapist or group?

_____ 57. Do you remain silent about your problems in group, rationalizing that the problems of others are more serious or important than yours?

_____ 58. Are you actively working to build a strong social support network of nondrug friends?

_____ 59. Are you immersed in guilt about your past behavior and thereby less able to focus on your present behavior in recovery?

_____ 60. Are you resisting the necessity to change your lifestyle?

_____ 61. Do you continue to experience frequent drug urges and cravings?

_____ 62. When you get a craving or urge do you tend to feel that your recovery is failing?

_____ 63. Do you fantasize about being able to return to using drugs in the future?

_____ 64. When not at work, do you tend to be idle and alone alot?

_____ 65. Do you feel resentful, self-conscious, or self-pitying about not drinking at restaurants, social gatherings, or business meetings?

_____ 66. Do you have a specific action plan for dealing with cravings and urges?

_____ 67. Are you reluctant to reach out for help from your group members or others for fear that they will perceive you as imperfect and weak?

_____ 68. Have you contacted anyone in your group for social reasons or support?

_____ 69. If you have a relapse, are you likely to leave treatment because of extreme embarrassment and feelings of failure?

_____ 70. Do you quietly resent being called an addict or alcoholic?

_____ 71. Do you get urges and cravings as a result of attending groups sessions or 12-step meetings?

_____ 72. Do you blame your drug use on a bad marriage, job stress, financial difficulties, or other major problems in your life?

_____ 73. Are you afraid to remain abstinent long enough to find out more about yourself and why you use drugs?

_____ 74. Do you feel that most of your problems would be solved if other people got off your case and treated you with more understanding?

_____ 75. Do you find yourself wanting to prove your therapist and peers wrong?

_____ 76. Do you believe that only someone who is a recovering addict is capable of understanding your problem and helping you with it?

_____ 77. Are you more focused on differences rather than similarities with other recovering addicts?

_____ 78. Are you resentful and angry about the investment of money and time you must devote to your recovery?

_____ 79. Do you tend to think that your treatment program is just a money-making scheme and that your therapist doesn't really care what happens to you?

_____ 80. Do you secretly mistrust your therapist and feel the need to control your treatment plan as much as possible?

_____ 81. Are you upset and disappointed when the group does not give priority to your issues and problems?

_____ 82. Do you feel competitive and resentful toward peers who are farther along in recovery than you are?

_____ 83. Are you left frustrated and angry when not provided with an immediate, concrete solution to a pressing problem you bring up in a group meeting or therapy session?

_____ 84. Are you intolerant of recovering peers who fail to agree with you?

_____ 85. Do you believe that having an addictive disease means that you have no control over whether or not you use drugs again?

_____ 86. Do you feel doomed to relapse and failure?

_____ 87. Are you "all talk and no action" when it comes to making the fundamental lifestyle and attitude changes that are necessary for your recovery?

_____ 88. Do you spend too much time dwelling on the faults of others?

_____ 89. Are you too defensive to take an honest personal inventory of your own shortcomings and mistakes?

_____ 90. Do you have a negative, pessimistic attitude about improving your life?

_____ 91. Are you resentful that some problems have actually gotten worse since you've stopped using drugs?

_____ 92. Are you living in a "pink cloud", believing that most problems are behind you?

_____ 93. Are you angry at others for confronting you about your drug-related behavior?

_____ 94. Do you fear that your recovery is going to be an intolerable experience?

_____ 95. Do you have rapid mood swings?

_____ 96. Do you tend to overreact to stressful situations?

_____ 97. Are you unproductive and chronically bored or distracted at work?

_____ 98. Are you chronically irritable, short-tempered, or argumentative?

_____ 99. If something especially *good* happened to you, would you be tempted to get high as a way of celebrating?

_____ 100. Are you alert for early warning signs of relapse and what to do about them in order to avoid returning to drugs?

APPENDIX H

Family Questionnaire

Part 1: GENERAL INFORMATION

1. Your name: _____   _____
   (last)   (first)
2. Name of primary patient _____
2. Today's date: _____ Your Age: _____
3. Referred by: _____
4. Your occupation: _____
5. Your employer: _____
6. Your home address: _____

   _____

7. Your home phone #: _____
8. Your office phone #: _____
9. Your relationship to the substance abuser: _____
10. Is he/she currently in treatment? _____
    If so, where? _____
11. How long have you known him/her? _____
12. Do you currently live with the patient and if so, for how long?

    _____

13. What recent crisis led you and/or the substance abuser to seek professional help? Please be specific.

    _____

    _____

    _____

Part 2: DESCRIPTION OF THE PROBLEM

Answer these questions to the best of your knowledge. *Please do not leave any blanks*. Where appropriate, write "don't know".

1. What are the patient's primary drug(s) of choice?
    _____

2. Check off below the substances that the patient has been using recently (within past 3 months) and whether his/her use of each substance is occasional, frequent, or compulsive.

	occasional	frequent	compulsive
___ Cocaine *snorting, smoking, injecting*	___	___	___
___ Alcohol *beer, wine, liquor*	___	___	___
___ Tranquilizers *valium, xanax, librium, etc.*	___	___	___
___ Sleeping Pills *seconol, tuinol, etc.,*	___	___	___
___ Pain Pills *codeine, fiurinol, percodan, demerol, etc.,*	___	___	___
___ Heroin	___	___	___
___ Marijuana	___	___	___
___ Hallucinogens *LSD, PCP, etc.,*	___	___	___
___ Inhalants *nitrous oxide, etc.,*	___	___	___
___ Anti-depressants *Norpramin, Tofranil, Elavil, Triavil, etc.,*	___	___	___
___ Other pills (specify)	___	___	___

3. Check off the *symptoms* and *consequences* associated with the patient's drug/alcohol problem.
    ___ personality changes _____
    ___ extreme & rapid mood swings _____
    ___ temper outbursts _____
    ___ extreme irritability _____
    ___ "blackouts" (memory loss) _____
    ___ fits of anger & rage _____
    ___ defensive & argumentative _____
    ___ secretive & socially withdrawn _____
    ___ lying and deceitful _____
    ___ physically abusive _____

_____ verbally abusive _____

_____ sexually abusive _____

_____ totally self-centered _____

_____ irrational & out-of-control behavior _____

_____ financial problems _____

_____ family problems _____

_____ health problems _____

_____ neglect of household chores _____

_____ neglect of parenting responsibilities _____

_____ neglect of work responsibilities _____

_____ legal problems _____

_____ loss of job, income _____

_____ loss of personal property _____

_____ isolation from family, friends, etc _____

_____ other _____

4. In addition to substance abuse, does the patient have problems with:

   a. _____ compulsive gambling
   b. _____ compulsive sexuality
   c. _____ compulsive eating (overeating, binging)
   d. _____ compulsive non-eating (fasting, anorexia)
   e. _____ workaholism
   f. _____ severe depression
   g. _____ suicidal thoughts
   h. _____ suicide attempts
   i. _____ violent behavior
   j. _____ hearing voices
   k. _____ bizarre thoughts/hallucinations
   l. _____ criminal behavior

5. In what settings does the patient use drugs/alcohol?
   Check all that apply:

   _____ in bars   _____ with co-workers
   _____ at work   _____ with friends
   _____ at home   _____ with spouse
   _____ in after-hours clubs   _____ with lover(s)
   _____ daily   _____ with you
   _____ on weekends only   _____ alone
   _____ in binges

6. For how long has the drug/alcohol problem existed?

   _____

7. *When* and *how* did you first become aware of the problem?

   _____

   _____

9. Please describe the patient's previous treatment for substance abuse and/or psychiatric problems.

   Hospitalizations: _____

   _____

   Outpatient Drug/Alcohol Programs _____

   _____

   Psychotherapy _____

   _____

   Other _____

   _____

10. If previous treatment for the substance abuse problem was *not* successful, describe why you think it did not yield better results. What do you think should be done *now* that was not done before, to improve success.

    Reasons for previous failure: _____

    _____

    _____

    What should be done now: _____

    _____

    _____

Part 3: IMPACT ON YOU AND THE FAMILY

1. In what ways have you tried to handle the patient's drug/alcohol problem? *Check all that apply.*

   _____ beg & plead   _____ nag & scream
   _____ fight & argue   _____ lecture & preach
   _____ "silent" treatment   _____ make idle threats
   _____ keep track of his/her   _____ pay bill/debts
         whereabouts   _____ buy food, clothing, etc
   _____ supply cash/credit cards   _____ keep him/her confined
   _____ pay other living expenses   _____ extend loans/credit
   _____ threaten users/dealers   _____ make excuses to boss
   _____ wakeup calls for work   _____ cover up/lie to others
   _____ bail out of legal trouble
   _____ taken over other responsibilities for the patient
   _____ go on search missions or send others to find him/her
   _____ play therapist/"shrink" trying to explain the problem
   _____ play "if you really loved me, you would stop" routine
   _____ play "if you don't stop, I'll get sick and die" routine
   _____ hide or discard drugs/alcohol/paraphernalia
   _____ leave temporarily, but always come back
   _____ call police/obtain order of protection

____ separation/divorce proceedings
____ counseling/therapy for yourself
____ attend Al-Anon, Coc-Anon or Nar-Anon self-help meetings
____ have thrown him/her out of the house
____ have cut off all financial assistance
____ have completely stopped trying to help
____ have been calling clinics/hospitals/doctors for help
____ other (please describe) _____

2. Which (if any) of the above things have helped in terms of getting the patient to acknowledge the problem and the need for help?
_____
_____
_____

3. How much money have you and/or other family members given the patient during the past month? $ _____
6 months? $ _____

4. Please give us *your* own personal view of the patient's drug/alcohol problem by answering the questions below.
a. In my view, the patient's drug/alcohol problem is:
____ mild　　____ moderate　　____ severe
b. The patient's drug/alcohol problem is an "illness" or "disease" requiring treatment and total abstinence.
____ true　　____ false
c. The patient's drugs/alcohol problem is just a symptom of his/her psychological problems.
____ true　　____ false
e. The drug/alcohol problem would stop if s/he would just change friends, job, or mate.
____ true　　____ false

5. In what ways has the patient's substance abuse problem caused problems for *you* and *your family?* Please check off and describe all that apply.
____ your emotional/mental state _____
____ your moods _____
____ your personality _____
____ your marital satisfaction _____
____ your sexuality _____
____ your financial status _____
____ your social life _____
____ your relationship w. others _____
____ your children _____

____ your job/career _____

____ your physical health _____

____ your physical appearance _____

____ your use of alcohol/drugs _____

____ your sleeping patterns _____

____ your eating patterns _____

____ the mood & atmosphere in your home _____

____ your hopes, fears, & worries _____

____ your general outlook on life _____

____ other _____

6. Which of the following problems are *you* experiencing?
   Check all that apply.

   ____ mental exhaustion   ____ depression

   ____ crying spells   ____ short temper

   ____ excessive sleeping   ____ insomnia

   ____ loss of sex drive   ____ excessive eating

   ____ loss of appetite   ____ poor attention span

   ____ digestion problems   ____ headaches

   ____ mood swings   ____ emotional outbursts

   ____ muscle/back pain   ____ chest pains

   ____ heart palpitations   ____ dizzy spells

7. What feelings does the patient's drug/alcohol use set off in *you*? Check
   all that apply.

   ____ anger/rage   ____ resentment   ____ disgust

   ____ hopelessness   ____ helplessness   ____ inadequacy

   ____ sorrow   ____ humiliation   ____ embarrassment

   ____ self-blame   ____ guilt   ____ contempt

   ____ indifference   ____ revenge   ____ disappointment

   ____ frustration   ____ compassion   ____ protectiveness

   ____ shame   ____ confusion   ____ inferiority

   ____ other _____
   _____

8. What do you think will happen to *you*, if the patient continues or
   returns to drugs/alcohol?

   _____

   _____

   _____

Part 4: MORE ABOUT YOU

1. Describe your own pattern of alcohol use.

   _____

   _____

2. What other mood-altering drugs (prescription or non-prescription) do you use?

Name of Drug	Amt/Freq of Use	Reasons for Use
_____	_____	_____
_____	_____	_____
_____	_____	_____
_____	_____	_____

3. Have you or others ever been concerned about *your* use of alcohol or drugs? If yes, please describe below.

_____

4. Have you ever sought treatment for alcohol/drug use? If yes, please give details below, including name of doctor/facility and dates of treatment.

_____

_____

5. Have you ever been involved in a self-help group for alcohol, drugs, eating, gambling, or smoking problems. If yes, give details below.

_____

6. Have you ever sought counseling/therapy for a psychological, family, marital, or other personal problem? If yes, give details below including type of problem, name of therapist/facility, and dates of treatment.

_____

_____

7. Answer the following questions about yourself as TRUE or False.
   _____ I adapt easily to difficult situations.
   _____ I rarely rely on the help of others.
   _____ I have difficulty saying "no" to requests for my help, even when I know I *should* say "no".
   _____ I devote more time and energy to solving the problems of others than to solving my own problems.
   _____ I easily take on other people's pain.
   _____ I overreact to situations over which I have no control.
   _____ I tend to judge myself without mercy.
   _____ I constantly seek the approval of others.
   _____ I am super responsible.
   _____ I am extremely loyal, even when it is undeserved.
   _____ I expend excessive energy cleaning up other people's mess.

_____ I have a history of being involved with other people who have substance abuse problems.

_____ I often feel responsible for the happiness of others.

_____ I would rather give in than make someone angry.

_____ If I stopped being so involved in the problems of others, I might have to face my own problems.

_____ I continue to believe that somehow I will be able to stop the substance abuser from hurting him/herself.

_____ If I stop helping the substance abuser, s/he will probably end up dead.

_____ I think that my attempts to "help" the substance abuser are useless and may even be making the problem worse.

_____ I feel like a hostage to the substance abuser's problem, but I can't let go.

8. Has any relative of yours (including parents, children, grandparents, siblings, aunts, uncles, etc.) ever had a problem with alcohol, drugs, or gambling? If yes, please give details below.

Relative	Problem	Ever Treated?

Bibliography

Blume, S. (1987). Alcohol problems in cocaine abusers. In A. M. Washton, & M. S. Gold (Eds.), *Cocaine: A clinician's handbook* (pp. 202–206). New York: Guilford.

Blume, S. B., & Lesieur, H. R. (1987). Pathological gambling in cocaine abusers. In A. M. Washton, & M. S. Gold (Eds.), *Cocaine: a clinician's handbook* (pp. 208–213). New York: Guilford.

Carnes, P. (1983). *Out of the shadows: Understanding sexual addiction*. Minneapolis: CompCare.

Chasnoff, L. J., & Schnoll, S. H. (1987). Consequences of cocaine and other drug use in pregnancy. In A. M. Washton, & M.S. Gold (Eds.), *Cocaine: A clinician's handbook* (pp. 241–246). New York: Guilford.

Cohen, S. (1985). *The substance abuse problems. Vol. 2. New issues for the 1980's*. New York: Haworth.

Cohen, S. (1987). Causes of the cocaine outbreak. In A. M. Washton, & M. S. Gold (Eds.), *Cocaine: A clinician's handbook* (pp. 3–8). New York: Guilford.

Cohen, S. (1988). *The chemical brain: The neurochemistry of addictive disorders*. Irvine: CareInstitute.

Estroff, T. W. (1987). Medical and biological complications of cocaine abuse. In A. M. Washton, & M. S. Gold (Eds.), *Cocaine: A clinician's handbook* (pp. 23–32). New York: Guilford.

Extein, I., & Dackis, C. A. (1987). Brain mechanisms in cocaine dependency. In A. M. Washton, & M. S. Gold (Eds.), *Cocaine: A clinician's handbook* (pp. 73–82). New York: Guilford.

Gold, M. S., Galanter, M., & Stimmel, B. (Eds.) (1987). *Cocaine: Pharmacology, addiction, and therapy*. New York: Haworth.

Gorski, T., & Miller, M. (1986). *Staying sober: A guide for relapse prevention*. Independence Mo: Independence Press.

Grabowski, J. (Ed.). (1984). *Cocaine: Pharmacology, effects, and treatment of abuse*. Washington DC: US Government Printing Office, DHHS publication number (ADM)84-601074.

Jones, R. T. (1987). Psychopharmacology of cocaine. In A. M. Washton, & M. S. Gold (Eds.), *Cocaine: A clinician's handbook* (pp. 55–67). New York: Guilford.

Khantzian, E. J. (1987). Psychiatric and psychodynamic factors in cocaine dependence. In

237

A.M. Washton, & M. S. Gold (Eds.), *Cocaine: A clinician's handbook* (pp. 229–240). New York: Guilford.

Kleber, H. D., & Gawin, F. H. (1987). Pharmacological treatments of cocaine abuse. In A. M. Washton, & M. S. Gold (Eds.), *Cocaine: A clinician's handbook* (pp. 118–131). New York: Guilford.

Lesieur, H. R., & Blume, S. B. (1987). The South Oaks Gambling Screen (SOGS): A new instrument for the identification of pathological gamblers. *American Journal of Psychiatry, 144*(9), 1184–1188.

Marlatt, G. A., & Gordon, J. R. (1985). *Relapse prevention*. New York: Guilford.

Morehouse, E. (1987). Treating adolescent cocaine abusers. In A. M. Washton, & M. S. Gold (Eds.), *Cocaine: A clinician's handbook* (pp. 135–150). New York: Guilford.

Siegel, R. K. (1987). Cocaine smoking: Nature and extent of coca paste and cocaine free-base abuse. In A. M. Washton, & M. S. Gold (Eds.), *Cocaine: A clinician's handbook* (pp. 175–191). New York: Guilford.

Snyder, S. H. (1986). *Drugs and the brain*. New York: Scientific American Books.

Spitz, H. I., & Rosecan, J. S. (1987). *Cocaine abuse: New directions in treatment and research*. New York: Brunner/Mazel.

Stone, N., Fromme, M., & Kagan, D. (1984). *Cocaine: Seduction and solution*. New York: Clarkson N. Potter.

Verebey, K. (1987). Cocaine abuse detection by laboratory methods. In A. M. Washton, & M. S. Gold (Eds.), *Cocaine: A clinician's handbook* (pp. 214–226). New York: Guilford.

Washton, A. M. (1987). Outpatient treatment techniques. In A. M. Washton, & M. S. Gold (Eds.), *Cocaine: A clinician's handbook* (pp. 106–117). New York: Guilford.

Washton, A. M. (1986, March). Women and cocaine. *Medical Aspects of Human Sexuality* (p. 57).

Washton, A. M. (1986, July 3). It's dangerous myth that cocaine is safe. *USA Today*. (guest editorial).

Washton, A. M. (1986, September). Crack. *Medical Aspects of Human Sexuality* (pp. 49–51).

Washton, A. M. (1988, February). Preventing relapse to cocaine. *Journal of Clinical Psychiatry, 49*, (Suppl. Vol. 2) 34–38.

Washton, A. M. (1987). Structured outpatient treatment of cocaine abuse. *Advance in Alcohol and Substance Abuse, 6*, 143–158.

Washton, A. M., & Boundy, D. (1989). *When willpower's not enough*. New York: Harper & Row.

Washton, A. M., & Boundy, D. (1989). *Cocaine and crack: What you need to know*. Hillsdale NJ: Enslow.

Washton, A. M., & Gold, M. S. (1984). Chronic cocaine abuse: Evidence for adverse effects on health and functioning. *Psychiatric Annals, 14*, 733–743.

Washton, A. M., & Gold, M. S. (1986). Crack. *Journal of the American Medical Association, 256*, 711.

Washton, A. M., & Gold, M. S. (1987). Recent trends in cocaine abuse as seen from the "800-Cocaine" Hotline. In A. M. Washton, & M. S. Gold (Eds.), *Cocaine: A clinician's handbook* (pp. 10–19). New York: Guilford.

Washton, A. M., Gold, M. S., & Pottash, A. L. C. (1983). Intranasal cocaine addiction. *Lancet, 2*, 1374.

Washton, A. M., Gold, M. S., Pottash, A. L. C., & Semlitz, L. (1984). Adolescent cocaine abusers. *Lancet, 2*, 746.

Washton, A. M., Gold, M. S., & Pottash, A. L. C. (1986). Crack: Early report on a new drug epidemic. *Postgraduate Medicine, 80*, 52–58.

Washton, A. M., Hendrickson, E., & Stone, N. (1988). Clinical assessment of the cocaine abuser. In Donovan, D., & Marlatt, G. A. (Eds.), *Assessment of addictive behaviors*. New York: Guilford.

Washton, A. M., & Tatarsky, A. (1984). Adverse effects of cocaine abuse. In L. S. Harris (Ed.), *Problems of drug dependence* (pp. 247–254). NIDA Research Monograph (No. 44). Washington DC: US Gov't Printing Office.

Weiss, R. D., & Mirin, S. M. (1987). *Cocaine*. Washington DC: American Psychiatric Press.

Wetli, C. V. (1987). Fatal reactions to cocaine. In A. M. Washton, & Gold, M.S. (Eds.), *Cocaine: A clinician's handbook* (pp. 33–50). New York: Guilford.

Index

239